THE EVERYTHING®
GUIDE TO MANAGING AND REVERSING PRE-DIABETES

Dear Reader,

The news that you have pre-diabetes is something you should take seriously. Whether you have just heard this news, or you have known for a while, you probably realize that healthy eating and lifestyle changes are necessary parts of your future. *The Everything® Guide to Managing and Reversing Pre-Diabetes* is a resource designed to help you make the transition to a healthier lifestyle and way of eating.

As a dietitian and diabetes educator in private practice, I've had many new clients come to my office who have just learned they have pre-diabetes. Invariably there is much confusion over the question "What can I eat?" There is often anticipation of hearing that favorite foods are going to be taken away. After we discuss what pre-diabetes is and how to make healthy eating and lifestyle choices, most of my clients leave their first appointments feeling pleasantly surprised. They have learned that managing pre-diabetes is about common sense and moderation, not deprivation.

The Everything® Guide to Managing and Reversing Pre-Diabetes provides you with vital information about the condition, and it has a large selection of recipes to help you start eating healthier. Cooking to manage pre-diabetes does not mean that separate meals or foods need to be made. The recipes and cooking methods described in this book provide healthy options for everyone in your household.

It is my sincere hope that the information in this book helps you on your path to managing your pre-diabetes. Your perseverance and follow through with the recommendations may make it possible to reverse the pre-diabetes. Taking action is the first step toward halting the progression of pre-diabetes.

For me, developing and testing the recipes found in this book has been a very enjoyable extension of my work as a Certified Diabetes Educator. When recipes result in great tasting foods, cooking becomes a pleasure. I hope you will come away feeling pleasantly surprised!

Gretchen Scalpi, RD, CDN, CDE

Welcome to the EVERYTHING® Series!

These handy, accessible books give you all you need to tackle a difficult project, gain a new hobby, comprehend a fascinating topic, prepare for an exam, or even brush up on something you learned back in school but have since forgotten.

You can choose to read an *Everything*® book from cover to cover or just pick out the information you want from our four useful boxes: e-questions, e-facts, e-alerts, and e-ssentials.

We give you everything you need to know on the subject, but throw in a lot of fun stuff along the way, too.

We now have more than 400 *Everything*® books in print, spanning such wide-ranging categories as weddings, pregnancy, cooking, music instruction, foreign language, crafts, pets, New Age, and so much more. When you're done reading them all, you can finally say you know *Everything*®!

QUESTION

Answers to
common questions

FACT

Important snippets
of information

ALERT

Urgent
warnings

ESSENTIAL

Quick
handy tips

PUBLISHER Karen Cooper

DIRECTOR OF ACQUISITIONS AND INNOVATION Paula Munier

MANAGING EDITOR, EVERYTHING® SERIES Lisa Laing

COPY CHIEF Casey Ebert

ASSISTANT PRODUCTION EDITOR Jacob Erickson

ACQUISITIONS EDITOR Katrina Schroeder

EDITORIAL ASSISTANT Ross Weisman

EVERYTHING® SERIES COVER DESIGNER Erin Alexander

LAYOUT DESIGNERS Colleen Cunningham, Elisabeth Lariviere, Ashley Vierra, Denise Wallace

THE EVERYTHING GUIDE TO MANAGING AND REVERSING PRE-DIABETES

Your complete plan for
preventing the onset of diabetes

Gretchen Scalpi, RD, CDN, CDE
Foreword by Robert Vigersky, MD

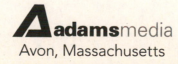

Avon, Massachusetts

*To my all of my clients with pre-diabetes
and diabetes who have taught me about challenges
and rewards of managing their health.*

An Everything® Series Book.
Everything® and everything.com® are registered trademarks of F+W Media, Inc.

Published by Adams Media, a division of F+W Media, Inc.
57 Littlefield Street, Avon, MA 02322 U.S.A.
www.adamsmedia.com

Contains material adapted and abridged from *The Everything® Diabetes
Cookbook, 2nd Edition* by Gretchen Scalpi, © 2010 by F+W Media, Inc.,
ISBN 10: 1-44050-154-8, ISBN 13: 978-1-44050-154-8.

ISBN 10: 1-4405-0985-9
ISBN 13: 978-1-4405-0985-8
eISBN 10: 1-4405-1077-6
eISBN 13: 978-1-4405-1077-9

Printed in the United States of America.

10 9 8 7 6 5 4 3 2 1

Library of Congress Cataloging-in-Publication Data
Scalpi, Gretchen.
The everything guide to managing and reversing pre-diabetes / Gretchen Scalpi.
p. cm.
Includes index.
1. Prediabetic state. I. Title.
RC660.S28   2011
616.4'62—dc22   2010041442

*This book is available at quantity discounts for bulk purchases.
For information, please call 1-800-289-0963.*

Contents

Acknowledgments

Thank you to the staff at Adams Media, especially Katrina Schroeder and Brett Shanahan, for their advice, encouragement, and technical support.

I am deeply appreciative to my husband John, who, for thirty-six years has supported my career endeavors, and always strived to make my life easier during busy and stressful times.

A special thanks to my dear friend Jon Hines, his wonderfully creative ideas, great food, good times, and everlasting friendship.

Foreword

As a practicing endocrinologist, I regularly see patients who have been ravaged by the dreaded complications of diabetes—blindness, amputations, kidney failure, and heart disease. These patients are taking an average of eight medications a day (one of which is often insulin) in order to control their blood sugar and its commonly associated conditions of high blood pressure and high cholesterol. Their lives and lifestyles (and those of their loved ones) have been permanently altered. Much of this could have been avoided if, instead of taking the ostrich approach to their health, they had taken the advice that their healthcare providers gave years earlier when they had pre-diabetes. Gretchen Scalpi has written a compelling and lucid account of the causes and management of pre-diabetes that makes it both easy and enjoyable to engage in the "ounces of prevention" that it takes to stay healthy. A book that helps you tackle this important personal health (and public health) issue couldn't be timelier since it is predicted that one of every three Americans born today will develop diabetes as an adult unless we find a way to stem this epidemic. Moreover, the advice in this book is applicable to even those who don't yet have pre-diabetes because the risk for developing diabetes (and cardiovascular disease) increases continuously from blood sugars as low as 80mg/dl—levels which may exist for years before the diagnosis of pre-diabetes (fasting blood sugar of 100–125mg/dl) or diabetes (fasting blood sugar of 126 or greater) are actually "official." This explains why even some patients who are newly diagnosed with diabetes already have some diabetic complications—they have had years of exposure to sugars that are physiologically abnormal despite what the laboratory's "normal range" is showing.

Strategies to improve one's lifestyle are essential to the prevention and/or delay of diabetes particularly since there are no medications that are approved for this purpose. Such strategies, which have been proven in large clinical trials to be effective in delaying the onset of diabetes, are laid out in a very practical and easily understandable format in this book. It is quite appropriate that Chapter 4 on exercise precedes a chapter on diet management since there is accumulating evidence that exercise not only burns off calories while you are doing it but also stimulates your cells to turn on their metabolism and burn sugar for hours afterward giving you "more bang for the buck." There are many useful tips on how to get started with an exercise program in Chapter 4 but one that should hit home to many is the advice to avoid buying a piece of exercise equipment at the outset. I have always fantasized that in retirement I'll open a used exercise equipment store stocked with my patients' bicycles, weight machines, etc., that were used enthusiastically for a few weeks but ultimately ended up as expensive clothes hangers or just dust collectors. Start simply and cheaply. Make a commitment in your time before you unnecessarily spend your hard-earned money. Chapter 5 is no less important in providing a sensible approach to choosing the right foods whether eating at home or in a restaurant. The bonus is that there are delicious recipes that apply the principles of these healthy choices. As a diabetes educator, Ms. Scalpi clearly believes that knowledge is power. Read this book and take advantage of your acquired power to stay healthy!

—Robert A. Vigersky, MD
Director, Diabetes Institute of the Walter Reed Health Care System
Past-President of The Endocrine Society

Introduction

IF YOU ARE READING this book, odds are that you have concerns about the fact that you or a loved one has pre-diabetes. Pre-diabetes often has no symptoms; therefore one may not realize he has the condition. Many of us know that we need to "do something" about our weight or lack of exercise, but until something goes wrong there seems no need for urgency. Once you have learned that you or a loved one has pre-diabetes, however, there is an urgency to take action.

Managing pre-diabetes means understanding what it is and what to do about it. The more you understand, the better you can take action to reverse it or minimize your risk of developing type 2 diabetes. Luckily, by reading this book and putting some ideas into practice, you will have taken the first steps toward learning all you can about managing and reversing pre-diabetes.

Before we delve into the specifics of pre-diabetes, here's a quick overview of diabetes. Once you understand more about diabetes, you will see the connection to pre-diabetes and why action on your part should not be put off.

DIABETES MELLITUS

Every time we eat, our body converts the foods we consume into glucose (sugar). Insulin is a hormone the body makes that enables the glucose to get into cells, and the glucose is used for energy. People with diabetes either lack sufficient amounts of insulin or are unable to use the insulin they make. When insulin is absent or ineffective, the body is unable to get energy into cells and the level of glucose in the blood increases. To put it simply, your blood sugar level is too high. Genetics, obesity, and lack of exercise appear to be causal factors in most cases of diabetes. There are different types of diabetes as well.

Type 1 Diabetes

Approximately 5–10 percent of known cases of diabetes are classified as type 1 diabetes. Type 1 diabetes was formerly referred to as juvenile-onset diabetes because the onset typically occurs before the age of thirty. Type 1 diabetes is an autoimmune disorder that is thought to develop when stress factors (such as a viral infection) damage or destroy the beta cells of the pancreas. The person with type 1 diabetes is always dependent upon insulin because their pancreas no longer produces insulin. Type 1 diabetes is usually not associated with obesity or lack of exercise. Our discussion of pre-diabetes in this book will be focused on type 2 diabetes rather than type 1 diabetes.

Type 2 Diabetes

Type 2 diabetes makes up the vast majority of individuals who have diabetes. For most people with type 2 diabetes, the pancreas still produces insulin, but it is being produced in insufficient amounts, or the body simply is unable to use the insulin in an efficient way.

Most people with type 2 diabetes are diagnosed in mid to late adulthood. Unfortunately, with the growing prevalence of obesity among children, we are now seeing children and young adults with type 2 diabetes as well.

Type 2 diabetes is often related to a sedentary lifestyle and an overweight or obese status. It is important to understand that diabetes is a disease that will progress and while it can be controlled, it cannot be cured. Over time many people with type 2 diabetes may require oral medications and/or insulin to effectively treat and manage the disease. If untreated, a person with pre-diabetes may go on to develop type 2 diabetes.

Gestational Diabetes

Gestational diabetes is similar to type 2 diabetes because the body still makes insulin, however a hormone secreted by the placenta interferes with the action of insulin. The result is elevated blood glucose levels usually starting around the twenty-fourth to twenty-eighth week of the pregnancy. In most cases, a pregnant woman's blood glucose returns to normal after the delivery of the baby and the diabetes is gone. A woman who has had gestational diabetes in the past has an increased risk of developing Type 2 diabetes at a later time in her life, especially if she remains overweight or sedentary.

For the purposes of this book, our discussions about diabetes refer to type 2 diabetes. Although the cause of type 2 diabetes is not completely understood, we know from statistics that it is increasing in the United States and throughout the world at an alarming rate. The goal of this book is to keep you from becoming part of the diabetes statistics.

Managing diabetes and pre-diabetes is all about making lifestyle changes. The 7 Self-Care Behaviors listed below apply to those with pre-diabetes and diabetes.

7 SELF-CARE BEHAVIORS

The American Association of Diabetes Educators believe that utilizing principles of the 7 Self-Care Behaviors is an effective way to make positive changes in lifestyle:

1. **Healthy Eating:** Make healthy food choices, understand portion sizes, and learn the best times to eat.
2. **Being Active:** Include regular activity for overall fitness, weight management, and blood glucose control.
3. **Monitoring:** Daily self-monitoring of blood glucose to assess how food, physical activity, and medications are working.
4. **Taking Medication:** Understand how medications work and when to take them.
5. **Problem Solving:** Know how to problem solve. For example, a high or low blood glucose episode could require the ability to make a quick decision about food, activity, or medication.
6. **Reducing Risks:** Effective risk reduction behaviors such as smoking cessation and regular eye exams are examples of self-care that reduce risk of complications.
7. **Healthy Coping:** Good coping skills that deal with the challenges of diabetes help people stay motivated to keep their diabetes in control.

As you read this book, you will find practical tools to empower you to take control of your health. Taking control means having an effective action plan that you can live with and is achievable. With practical tools and an effective plan, you have been given an opportunity to prevent or delay the onset of type 2 diabetes. Take it!

CHAPTER 1

What Is Pre-Diabetes?

Your doctor has just told you that you or your loved one has pre-diabetes. Your initial reaction might have been shock, anger, or a feeling of helplessness. Perhaps you knew something was not quite right all along, but you had put off going to the doctor and tried to put the whole thing out of your mind. Whatever the case, you are now faced with a medical diagnosis that has the potential to be serious. Many people in this situation find that they have not been given any tangible instructions about what pre-diabetes means or what to do about it. Somehow tips like "just lose some weight" or "don't eat any carbs" sound easy, but exactly how do you accomplish those things? The best place to start is to learn more about pre-diabetes, then put together your action plan to stop pre-diabetes in its tracks.

The Pre-Diabetes Epidemic in America

The most recent data from the National Diabetes Fact Sheet states there are an estimated 57 million Americans with pre-diabetes. Yes, you read that correctly: 57 million Americans! The number of cases grows annually, in large part because the presence of pre-diabetes is linked to America's serious health problems: overweight and obesity. Being overweight and having elevated blood sugar (either diabetes or pre-diabetes) tend to go hand in hand. Blood sugar that fluctuates too high or too low throughout the day has a direct influence on your hunger level, snacking habits, and overeating. If your blood sugar is too low, you may eat too much food. If you eat too much food, over time you gain weight. When you gain too much weight, you are setting the stage for developing pre-diabetes, or worse yet, diabetes.

If you are obese, your risk for developing diabetes is far greater than for someone whose weight is normal. Today roughly 2 out of every 3 American adults are heavy enough to be considered overweight or obese. At the same time the percentage of Americans with diabetes has increased by more than 30 percent since the 1970s. One thing is very clear about this trend: it means that the number of people who will develop diabetes or pre-diabetes is going to continue to grow.

Who Is Affected by Diabetes or Pre-Diabetes?

According to a recent study from the National Institutes of Health and the Centers for Disease Control and Prevention, nearly 13 percent of adults age twenty and older have diabetes. Diabetes is especially common in the elderly; nearly one-third of those age sixty-five and older have the disease. An additional 30 percent of adults have pre-diabetes, a condition marked by elevated blood sugar that is not yet in the diabetic range.

Pre-diabetes is more common in men than in women (36 percent for men compared to 23 percent for women). About 16 percent of children ages twelve to nineteen years have pre-diabetes. These findings were reported in the February 2009 issue of *Diabetes Care*.

Our Younger Generations: What's Going On?

The media is filled with reports about the troubling increase of childhood and adolescent obesity. Obesity among children has been steadily increasing over the past three decades. Obesity rates have doubled for preschool children (aged two to five) and adolescents (aged twelve to nineteen). For elementary children (aged six to eleven) the obesity rate has tripled since 1980. Today, overweight school-age children have become the norm, whereas several decades ago, overweight or obese children were much less common.

FACT

The prevalence of diabetes, diagnosed and undiagnosed, in non-Hispanic blacks and Mexican Americans is disproportionately higher (70 to 80 percent) than in non-Hispanic whites. The breakdown is: Non-Hispanic Whites: 29 percent; Non-Hispanic Blacks: 25 percent; and Mexican Americans: 32 percent. (*Diabetes Care*, February 2009)

What are the key reasons for this alarming increase? There are several factors. Our food habits have changed a lot over that past several decades. Most of today's children have exposure to a vast array of fast foods, convenience foods, and empty-calorie snack foods. Tempting foods are readily available everywhere and at any time. Children learn about fast foods, soft drinks, and snacks through repeated exposure to television and other forms of advertising. Grocery store aisles are filled with sweetened foods, cereals, beverages, candies, and even kid-specific versions of yogurt with cookie and candy toppings. Food products are targeted and marketed specifically to children. A quick review of Saturday morning cartoons can teach you something about how products are pitched to children. It comes as no surprise that children want and request foods or snacks that have been heavily marketed to them.

In addition, today's families rely much more on eating out. Fast foods, convenience, or take-out foods are consumed often. Reasons for relying on this type of food vary from simply lacking the time or energy to plan healthy meals at home, to not understanding the importance to good nutrition. Parents want to do the right thing for their children, but fast-paced lifestyles have gotten in the way. For some, family dinner at home has been replaced by dinner in the car at the drive-through. Unfortunately, many children learn to make strong associations with foods and beverages that have little nutritional value and in fact contribute to obesity. Like adults, overweight or obese children are far more likely to develop pre-diabetes or type 2 diabetes.

What Makes Pre-Diabetes Different from Type 2 Diabetes?

The term *pre-diabetes* was introduced by the American Diabetes Association in 2002 as a way to more clearly convey a state that is between normal blood sugar and type 2 diabetes. In the past your doctor may have diagnosed you with "borderline diabetes." Other statements that have been used (euphemistically) are "your blood sugar is a little high" or "you have a touch of sugar." These words provide little meaning to the person hearing them and they certainly do not express the urgent need to do something about the situation. Pre-diabetes is defined by tangible parameters, namely the results of blood glucose tests:

- **Normal is defined as:** fasting blood glucose is less than 100mg/dl and a glucose level less than 140mg/dl two hours after eating.
- **Pre-diabetes is defined as:** fasting blood glucose between 100–125mg/dl and a glucose level between 140–190mg/dl two hours after eating.
- **Diabetes is defined as:** fasting blood glucose of 126mg/dl or higher or a blood glucose greater than 200mg/dl two hours after eating.

ESSENTIAL

To confirm a diagnosis of either pre-diabetes or diabetes, the blood glucose levels must be elevated and within defined lab results at least two times. If your lab results indicated high glucose readings during an initial test, your doctor should repeat the test a second time to see whether the results are the same.

When you have pre-diabetes, your blood sugar level is higher than normal, but it's not yet high enough to be classified as type 2 diabetes. Pre-diabetes means that you are on your way to developing diabetes if there are no interventions on your part. One very important fact to understand is that progressing to type 2 diabetes is *not* inevitable. There is a great deal that you can do to reverse pre-diabetes and bring your blood sugar level back to a normal range. A diagnosis of type 2 diabetes, on the other hand, is permanent. While there is much that can be done to *control* diabetes, it is important to realize that type 2 diabetes does not go away. In spite of every-thing you have read so far, if you have received a diagnosis of pre-diabetes there is some good news. You have received a wake-up call and been given an opportunity to improve your health, lose weight, and make healthy life-style changes. If you take action you can prevent, or at the very least, halt the progression to a serious, permanent disease.

Risk Factors and Symptoms

In addition to laboratory results for fasting and post-meal glucose levels, there are other risk factors to consider. The risk factors that increase your risk of type 2 diabetes are the same risk factors for pre-diabetes. Check to see whether you fit any of these:

- **Age:** 45 or older
- **Family History:** A parent or sibling with type 2 diabetes
- **Weight:** Overweight or obese (the *primary* risk factor for pre-diabetes)
- **Race/Ethnic Background:** Hispanic, American Indian, African-Ameri-can, Asian-American, and Pacific-Islander
- **Exercise:** Inactive and sedentary lifestyle
- **Pregnancy:** Gestational diabetes during a past pregnancy
- **Other Conditions:** Polycystic Ovary Syndrome (PCOS)
- **Other Conditions:** Inadequate sleep of fewer than 5.5 hours nightly

Risk factors are used to determine increased susceptibility. The more risk factors present in your profile, the greater the risk for developing pre-diabetes or diabetes.

What about Symptoms?

Symptoms associated with pre-diabetes can be nonexistent or indistin-guishable from other causes. Early symptoms of pre-diabetes are so com-mon in fact, that many people barely notice them at all, or think that what they are feeling is "normal." Most symptoms are vague, very common, and rarely interfere with daily activities. However, sometimes the red flags asso-ciated with type 2 diabetes begin to appear, such as:

- Increased thirst
- Frequent urination
- Fatigue that doesn't improve with more sleep
- Blurred vision that may come and go

It is often not until several symptoms are noticed that a person begins to realize that things are not quite right.

QUESTION

What is acanthosis nigricans?
Acanthosis nigicans is one of the few early signs of pre-diabetes and may be noticed by an individual. It is characterized by a darkened area of skin which typically affects the neck, armpits, elbows, knees or knuckles. The darkening of pigment around these areas of the body can be an early sign of glucose abnormality. It is sometimes seen in children with type 2 diabetes. The condition does not affect everyone, and it requires no specific treatment.

Why You Can't Ignore Pre-Diabetes

Not that long ago, doctors did not routinely screen for, or treat, pre-diabetes aggressively. People who had glucose readings that were higher than normal but were not yet diabetic seldom received advice to reduce their risk of developing type 2 diabetes. That was before there was a good understanding about how glucose levels in the pre-diabetic range could actually cause vascular damage or other complications. Today we know that waiting until someone has progressed to diabetes could mean that complications have already begun to take hold. For this reason, the fasting blood glucose cutoff for pre-diabetes was lowered from 140mg/dl to 125mg/dl. Today a normal fasting blood glucose cutoff is below 100mg/dl, down from a previous 110mg/dl. The lowering of the blood glucose ranges has helped detect poor glucose tolerance in many people, much earlier.

If you've been informed that you have pre-diabetes, you can be grateful that you know about the problem now, at an early stage. The most compelling reason for addressing pre-diabetes is being able to halt or slow the progression to diabetes. If the right things are done at an early stage, a person may be able to reverse the pre-diabetic state. Even if you are only able to slow down the eventual progression to diabetes, you can minimize your risk for developing diabetic complications, such as heart disease, kidney failure, and diabetic retinopathy.

ALERT

People who do nothing and allow their blood sugar to creep up over time may already be developing some of the complications associated with diabetes. According to the American Diabetes Association, some long-term damage to the body, especially the heart and circulatory system, may already be occurring during pre-diabetes. Taking actions early on can help you prevent diabetic complications.

It is important to understand that diabetes does not occur suddenly. For most people, the progression from normal to pre-diabetic then to diabetic can take a number of years. The longer your body experiences high glucose levels, the greater your chance of developing diabetes-related complications.

CHAPTER 2

Diagnosing Pre-Diabetes

If you are trying to determine whether you have pre-diabetes, or monitor your condition after you have been diagnosed, you will need to have some information about your health. This information includes lab tests, blood pressure and other measurements such as height, weight, and waist circumference. Your prior health history provides additional clues in the determination of pre-diabetes or diabetes.

Getting Tested and Understanding the Results

A fasting blood glucose test is the first essential test that provides a clue about the possibility of pre-diabetes. This is a simple blood test where a sample of blood is drawn first thing in the morning after an overnight fast. A fasting blood glucose between 100 and 125mg/dl on more than one occasion is an indicator for pre-diabetes. Some doctors prefer using a *glucose challenge* rather than a fasting test. In this case, you are given a glucose drink that provides 75g of glucose. Blood is drawn two hours after taking the drink and then the blood glucose is measured.

With this test, a blood glucose result of 140–199mg/dl two hours after taking 75g of glucose (on more than one occasion) indicates pre-diabetes. Two-hour readings that are above 200mg/dl on more than one occasion indicate diabetes.

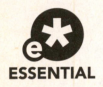

ESSENTIAL

A fasting blood glucose test means just that: fasting. If you are having your blood test in the morning you should not have anything to eat or drink (besides water) after midnight. Refrain from doing exercise before your test, because that could affect your reading, providing an inaccurate result.

What Other Blood Tests Are Important?

There are several other useful tests that can be helpful not only for determining pre-diabetes, but also for monitoring it once diagnosed.

When a fasting glucose test or two-hour glucose challenge is done, the reading provides a result for that moment in time. Because your glucose can vary a great deal throughout the day, these tests do not provide information about how your blood sugar is at other times of the day. That is why a test called the *hemoglobin A1c* is done, particularly when pre-diabetes or diabetes is suspected. Hemoglobin is a substance found in red blood cells which carries oxygen from the lungs to all cells in the body. When hemoglobin binds with glucose, an irreversible compound, *glycated hemoglobin* (or glycohemoglobin) is formed. The *A1c* portion of glycated hemoglobin is the easiest and largest portion of this compound to measure. A person with higher blood glucose has more glycated hemoglobin formed than someone with normal blood glucose. Hemoglobin found in red blood cells lasts for sixty to ninety days. As a result, when Hemoglobin A1c is measured, a fairly accurate reflection of your average blood glucose levels over the last sixty to ninety is determined. A hemoglobin A1c between 6–7 percent matches average glucose levels typically found in pre-diabetes. Monitoring your hemoglobin A1c and keeping it below 6 percent should be part of your action plan. Your doctor will monitor your hemoglobin A1c every three to six months by ordering a blood test.

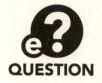
QUESTION

Do I need a glucose meter even if I don't have diabetes?
If you have been diagnosed with pre-diabetes, monitoring your own blood sugar with a glucose meter periodically can be a valuable tool to help you track your blood sugar. A glucose meter can be purchased over the counter or prescribed by your doctor. All meters come with easy to follow instructions. The readings from the glucose meter will help you learn how different foods affect your blood glucose, or what times of day you may be high or low. You can decide how often to check your blood glucose, but two to three times weekly may be a good start.

Cholesterol and Triglycerides

The relationship between cholesterol and heart disease is well known. People with pre-diabetes or diabetes have more risk for heart disease, therefore monitoring your cholesterol levels is an important part of your health plan. Knowing your total cholesterol is not sufficient to determine whether you are at risk. You also need to know how much of your total cholesterol represents good cholesterol (HDL) or bad cholesterol (LDL). Triglycerides, another type of fat found in the blood, is also associated with determining risk factors for heart disease. Below are recommended levels for cholesterol and triglyceride levels for individuals without diabetes or pre-diabetes. If you have pre-diabetes, you doctor may want to see readings even lower. The following list indicates normal laboratory values for cholesterol and triglycerides.

- **Total Cholesterol:** Less than 200mg/dl
- **LDL Cholesterol:** Less than 100mg/dl
- **HDL Cholesterol:** Greater than 40mg/dl for men; Greater than 50mg/dl for women
- **Triglycerides:** Less than 150mg/dl

LDL and HDL levels are much better predictors of heart disease risk than the total cholesterol. Although someone may have a normal total cholesterol reading, they can still be at increased risk if the LDL (bad) cholesterol is higher than recommended levels. If the results of your cholesterol or triglycerides are abnormal, you and your doctor will discuss these results. In addition to lab results, other risk factors such as gender, family history, smoking, weight, and blood pressure help determine the best course of treatment for you. For some individuals, healthy diet, modest weight loss, and a regular exercise plan may be enough to bring cholesterol and triglyceride levels in range. For others, the addition of cholesterol and/or triglyceride lowering medications may be necessary.

ESSENTIAL

The *lipid panel*, which measures total cholesterol, HDL, LDL, and triglycerides should be done at least annually. If your doctor has prescribed cholesterol or triglyceride lowering medications for you, a lipid panel, as well as other blood tests, may be required more often to monitor your body's response to the medication.

C-Reactive Protein (CRP)

C-Reactive Protein is a protein found in the blood, which indicates the amount of inflammation in your body. Inflammation plays a role in pre-diabetes and diabetes. A high-sensitive C-Reactive Protein (hsCRP) test can identify low-grade inflammation that increases one's risk for developing heart disease, making this a useful test for people at high risk for heart disease. Elevated CRP levels can also be found in some people with pre-diabetes, diabetes, or who are overweight.

Blood Pressure

Just as the prevalence of pre-diabetes and diabetes is on the rise, having hypertension (high blood pressure) is on the rise as well. Being overweight and having a sedentary lifestyle are two key reasons for an increased prevalence of high blood pressure. Sodium intake in one's diet can be a cause of high blood pressure. Although the recommendation for sodium intake is less than 2,400mg daily, many people consume much more sodium because they are using convenience, packaged, or processed foods often. Processed food accounts for a large percentage of the sodium Americans consume on a daily basis. A person who is *salt sensitive* may develop high blood pressure as a result of high sodium intake.

Blood pressure is the force of blood against the walls of arteries. The measurement is written one above the other, with the systolic number on top and the diastolic number on the bottom. Systolic blood pressure represents the force with which your heart pumps blood into the arteries. Diastolic blood pressure measures the pressure in the arteries when the heart is at rest, between heartbeats. High blood pressure needs to be treated because continued high pressure exerted on arteries can cause damage to the arteries or the heart.

The American College of Endocrinology (ACE) Task Force on the Prevention on Diabetes recommends a target blood pressure of 130/80 for persons with pre-diabetes. This is the same target for persons with diabetes.

About Metabolic Syndrome

Metabolic syndrome is a name used for a group of risk factors that, if present, increase your risk for having heart disease or other problems such as diabetes. Metabolic syndrome develops for many of the same reasons that pre-diabetes does. The treatment of metabolic syndrome is the same as for pre-diabetes. If you have a diagnosis of pre-diabetes, there may be a good chance that you have metabolic syndrome as well.

People who are overweight or obese and physically inactive are more likely to develop metabolic syndrome and insulin resistance. Having excess fat in the abdominal area, and a large waist circumference increases the likelihood of insulin resistance.

Insulin resistance is a condition where the body is unable to use its own insulin properly. Insulin, a hormone made by the pancreas, helps the body to use glucose for energy. People with insulin resistance require and may produce more insulin to help glucose get into cells. A consistent overproduction of insulin, coupled with overeating promotes weight gain. Eventually, the pancreas is no longer able to keep up with insulin demand and blood glucose begins to rise to the diabetic range.

ALERT

Metabolic syndrome means you have three or more conditions that together increase risk for heart disease, stroke, and diabetes. Specifically those conditions include: Large waist circumference (more than 36 inches in women and 40 inches in men), blood pressure higher than 130/85 mmHg, elevated triglyceride level and a low level of HDL cholesterol, and insulin resistance.

Family history and older age are other possible factors in metabolic syndrome. Obviously genetics and age cannot be controlled, however weight, blood fats, blood pressure, and blood glucose are factors that you can have influence over.

Women at Risk

Polycystic ovary syndrome (PCOS) is a grouping of reproductive health problems characterized by polycystic (many cysts) ovaries, irregular menstrual cycles, infertility, and obesity. Women with PCOS have *hyperinsulinism*, which means that high amounts of insulin are routinely produced. Like metabolic syndrome, an overproduction of insulin triggers a cycle of easy weight gain and insulin resistance. Some women with PCOS have metabolic syndrome. A woman with PCOS can have other symptoms such as acanthosis nigricans (dark skin patches), acne, facial hair, and loss of scalp hair. Lowering insulin levels and improving insulin sensitivity are the key strategies to managing PCOS. Without treatment of hyperinsulinism, weight gain and other metabolic abnormalities may occur. A woman with PCOS can go on to develop pre-diabetes or type 2 diabetes.

Treatment for PCOS is strikingly similar to treatment strategies used for pre-diabetes or metabolic syndrome. Weight loss, proper diet, and increased physical activity are considered essential components of treatment for PCOS. In some cases oral contraceptives to correct hormonal abnormalities and a medication such as Metformin (an insulin sensitizer used to treat diabetes) can improve symptoms associated with PCOS.

Pre-Diabetes and Overweight Kids

Being overweight or obese is the primary reason why children and adolescents are being diagnosed with pre-diabetes. Thirty years ago it was extremely uncommon to see a child with pre-diabetes. Today healthcare practitioners not only see children and adolescents with pre-diabetes, they diagnose and treat type 2 diabetes in this very population. Type 2 diabetes was once regarded as an adult-onset form of diabetes, and not a form of diabetes that affected children or adolescents. According to data from the 2007 National Diabetes Fact Sheet, approximately 2 million adolescents (or 1 in 6 overweight adolescents) have pre-diabetes.

QUESTION

My child has pre-diabetes. Does this mean he will develop type 2 diabetes?
Progressing from pre-diabetes to type 2 diabetes is *not* inevitable for children (or adults). The earlier pre-diabetes is addressed, the more possible it is to reverse. Children learn and copy parental behavior whether it's good or bad. If your child has pre-diabetes, help him get started with healthier lifestyle choices by setting a good example yourself.

Advances in medicine have contributed to the gradual increase in longevity for each successive generation. Now, however, this trend is about to change, and for the first time in decades, we can anticipate that today's children will develop health issues, chronic diseases, and complications at a much earlier age in life than their parents or grandparents. Earlier onset of chronic disease will mean a decline in the life expectancies of younger generations. The increased amount of obesity and pre-diabetes in our children will play a major role in this unfortunate development.

Pre-diabetes in children is determined in the same manner as in adults. Laboratory blood tests, and determination of overweight or obese status provide early clues of possible pre-diabetes. Like adults, treating pre-diabetes in children involves working on better lifestyle choices:

- Limiting fast foods, high-calorie, or empty-calorie foods and snacks
- Including more lower-calorie foods such as fruits and vegetables on a daily basis
- Getting physical activity for at least an hour every day
- Cutting down on TV or video-game time every day

The key to helping children make lifestyle changes is get them engaged and involved in the process. Letting children help with (safe) food preparation tasks in the kitchen, or asking them to go along grocery shopping to select healthy snacks are examples of how a child can be involved. The Alliance for a Healthier Generation (*www.healthiergeneration.org*) and Let's Move (*www.letsmove.gov*) are helpful websites offering practical ideas to help parents and their children work toward healthy lifestyle behaviors.

CHAPTER 3

Your Action Plan for Pre-Diabetes

By now you understand the potential consequences of untreated pre-diabetes. It is important to develop an action plan. Your action plan will help you make lifestyle changes gradually that will be implemented on a day-to-day basis. Have specific, tangible goals to work on. Generally, no more than two or three specific goals should be worked on at one time. This strategy prevents you from getting overwhelmed and allows you to master a goal before moving on to something else. Building in a small reward system for goals achieved can be a powerful way to keep you motivated. Rewards such a buying a new CD or book, going to a movie, or spending leisure time on a favorite hobby are examples of ways to celebrate progress.

Halting the Progression of Pre-Diabetes to Type 2 Diabetes

Halting the progression of pre-diabetes is extremely important and necessary to restore good health. With pre-diabetes, there is still a chance for you to reverse the progression and prevent onset of type 2 diabetes. Even if you develop diabetes eventually at a later time, slowing down the progression will result in fewer complications. Without taking action, progression to full-blown type 2 diabetes is a likely possibility.

There are three essential components to your action plan. First, most people with pre-diabetes will need to lose weight. Although you may know what it takes to lose weight, being consistent and keeping weight off is much more of a challenge than actually losing the weight. Second, you will need to work on gradual behavioral changes such as eating out less often or focusing on portion control. Third, you will need to begin and maintain a plan for routine exercise plan that is right for you.

Your Weight's Influence on Pre-Diabetes

Your weight may be only one of several causes for pre-diabetes, however, it is one factor that can you can control. Body Mass Index (BMI) is the primary way healthcare practitioners determine whether you are at a healthy weight, overweight, or obese. It is important to know your BMI. As you begin to lose weight, you can adjust and track your BMI.

BMI can be determined using a special BMI chart. If you do not a chart available, you can calculate your BMI in the following way:

1. Multiply your weight in pounds by 703.
2. Divide the result by your height in inches.
3. Divide this result by your height in inches again, and this will be your BMI.

A BMI of 18.5 to 24.9 is considered normal weight.
A BMI of 25 to 29.9 is considered overweight.
A BMI of 30 or greater is considered obese.

If you prefer to use a BMI calculator, go to *www.nhlbisupport.com/bmi*.

There are many rewards that come with weight loss. Research has shown that weight loss of as little as ten to twenty pounds can prevent or delay progression to diabetes. Even weight loss of a just few pounds will provide health benefits right away. Once you begin losing weight, insulin resistance will be reduced and insulin sensitivity will increase. This means that your blood glucose levels will be lower long before you reach you weight goal. Over time, weight loss can help reduce blood lipid (cholesterol and triglyceride) levels and lower blood pressure. For some, lower lipid levels or blood pressure can reduce the need for medication. An overall reduction in weight reduces the chances of having a heart attack, stroke, gallbladder disease, bone or joint problems, and certain types of cancer. Problems related to poor quality sleep, sleep apnea, and other breathing problems are known to improve with weight loss.

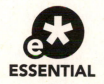

ESSENTIAL

Expecting that you will lose weight quickly is not realistic or long lasting. Losing a half to one pound a week over a period of time will go much further in helping you achieve results. Instead of focusing on a specific weight number on the scale, use positive observations to stay on track. Clothing that fits better or an increased energy level is a good way to gauge your progress. Whatever amount of weight you lose will be of benefit.

The point in time when modest weight loss is most likely to improve your health is when you have pre-diabetes or are in the very early stages of diabetes. Over time, persons with type 2 diabetes lose the ability to make adequate amounts of insulin. When this happens, weight loss and exercise alone are not enough to control blood glucose. Medications to lower blood glucose become a necessary part of treatment. Knowing that you may be able to avoid the need for medication is a good motivator for losing weight and keeping it off.

Facing Your Food Problems

You probably can identify certain food choices you make that need to be changed because of the ill affect they have on your health and weight. For some people it's salty snack foods, for others it may be ice cream or bakery items. Now is a good time to identify your problem foods and work on ways to reduce your exposure to them.

It's important to learn how to make your food environment safe and keep it as free as possible from foods that can cause problem eating and extra calories. Start by reviewing the foods you routinely buy at the grocery store weekly. Are these foods helping you reach your goals or are they self-sabotaging? What kinds of foods are in the cupboards or freezer? Many people have a hard time cleaning up their food environment because of other people living in the households. Keeping salty snacks or ice cream in the house because "the kids want them" is not likely to help you stay on track. Remember that healthy eating should be for everyone and having problem foods around the house constantly is going to make it difficult for anyone to resist eating these foods. Discuss your food problems with your family and come to some agreements regarding how often and how much of these foods should be allowed in the household. Help your family understand that if tempting, high-calorie foods are in the house all of the time, you are not going to be able to ignore them!

Foods that are sweet or salty taste good and temporarily make us feel good. The problem is, the immediate satisfaction we get from these foods is hard to pass up and in no time at all, we are back for more. Relying on will-power to stop you from eating irresistible foods will not work if faced with these food choices every day. In fact, willpower should not be one of your ongoing strategies to improve your eating habits. Make your food environment safer by keeping healthier food and snack alternatives available at all times. Remove your problem foods from the house on a regular basis and you will begin to move away from consuming these foods.

Of course, it is difficult (and for most, pretty impossible) to never eat the foods you love. If you decide *never* to eat a particular food, you may become obsessed with it and end up overeating it when given the opportunity. Instead, give yourself permission to have the food during a special occasion or celebration. Find a way to balance the problem food in a healthy way by not restricting, but rather reserving it for a certain time when you are free to really enjoy it. Lifelong healthy eating is about choice and finding a way to balance all the foods that you enjoy.

When you go grocery shopping, be sure to purchase a few healthy snack items. Many people find that if they have healthy snacks available, it becomes easier to use them in the absence of the high-calorie snacks. Availability of healthy food takes away the impulsiveness of poor food decisions.

Having one or two snacks during the day is a good way to keep you blood glucose stable and take the edge off your hunger. By using low-calorie snacks between meals, you can feel satisfied until your next meal. Try to keep your snacks in the range of 100–200 calories.

Here are a few examples of low-calorie snacks to have available in your safe food environment:

- Carrot sticks or sliced peppers with 2 tablespoons hummus for dipping
- Low-fat mozzarella cheese stick and a small apple
- 1 tablespoon peanut butter on 4 whole-grain crackers
- 6 ounces light or plain yogurt with a ¼ cup berries
- 10–12 nuts and a small piece of fruit of your choice

Get Moving (Every Day!)

Exercise has to be part of your action plan for halting pre-diabetes. The role of exercise cannot be underestimated or lacking from your overall plan. Before starting an exercise program decide what you can do and how to keep it as simple as possible. Too often, people become overenthusiastic at first, overdo it, and then burn out. Once this happens, they may not resume exercise at all. Start with one easy goal and master it for a few weeks before moving on to something else.

For some, the most difficult part of exercise is figuring out when they can fit it into their busy days. If this is you, try keeping a log of your daily activities for several days, then examine where there may be a small block of time to work in some exercise.

CHAPTER 4

Exercise: Essential for Your Success

Being more active is an important part of your pre-diabetes plan. Regular activity and exercise will improve your blood glucose levels. Lower blood glucose levels are achieved when the glucose in your blood is used for energy during and after exercise. Muscle cells become more sensitive to insulin, allowing for better storage and usage of glucose for energy. Cells in the liver also become more sensitive to insulin, and this helps prevent the liver from producing too much glucose. In essence, insulin resistance improves with regular exercise, and gradually blood glucose levels go down. Exercise has added benefits of strengthening your heart, helping to lower blood pressure, and helping with weight loss. Routine exercise is vital to the process of stopping pre-diabetes from progressing to diabetes, and improving your general health.

How Do I Get Started?

When you first learned about having pre-diabetes, your doctor probably encouraged you to begin exercising. If this was not initially discussed, you should talk to your doctor to make sure that exercise is appropriate for you. In most cases, your doctor will support your desire to start an exercise plan. If you have other health issues in addition to pre-diabetes, you and your doctor will want to discuss the best types of exercise for you. Be realistic when choosing exercises for yourself. Once your doctor has given you the okay to start, it's time to consider the variables that will help you choose the right type of exercise:

- Consider your ability to physically perform certain activities and choose activities that you can do. Some exercises may be too difficult or strenuous for your current level of fitness.
- Include activities you enjoy or those already performed on a regular basis. Going for a walk, gardening, or vacuuming are all activities that can easily help get you moving and be part of your daily routine.
- Think about how much time you have. An ambitious exercise plan that involves too much time will quickly be abandoned if you lack the time. If you have not exercised recently, ease into a program that includes short periods of time to start with.
- Consider the resources available to you. If you do not have access to a gym, exercise equipment, or a pool, then a simple walking plan may be your best bet.

ALERT

Resist the temptation to purchase home exercise equipment until you have tried it out and are reasonably sure that you will use it. Many types of home equipment end up at garage sales or just taking up space because the owner stopped using the equipment after a short period of time. If you are considering the purchase of home exercise equipment try it out first in the store, at a gym, or a friend's house before buying it. Make sure you like the activity enough that you will want to do it often!

When you make plans for exercise and activity, it is important to be honest about your likelihood to maintain the plan. Make sure to have activities that you will enjoy, or do not mind doing. Would you prefer to exercise alone or with the company of a friend or spouse? Will your activity involve being outdoors or indoors? Can you perform the activity outdoors year-round or will you need to find an alternate indoor activity for part of the year? Try to work out any barriers ahead of time that could get in the way of your exercise plan.

Making Time for Exercise

Your exercise routine should be planned to fit naturally into your daily schedule. Look at your daily routine, then decide where you can realistically fit in some time for activity. Short periods of time (ten to thirty minutes) will probably work much better than trying to carve out an hour for daily activity. Start out with small amounts of time one or more times of day. You will likely have more success getting in more activity this way. Here are a few examples of how you can slip in a little bit of activity every day without making huge demands on your schedule:

- Find opportunities to walk by arriving at your destination early, parking further away, then walking for ten minutes.
- During the work day, get up from your desk to walk around every hour. Take the stairs whenever you can and do this several times during the day.
- Go for a ten-minute walk after lunch or dinner.
- Spend ten minutes at the beginning and end of each day doing a few stretching exercises.
- Remember that many routine household activities such as cleaning, vacuuming, carrying groceries, gardening, and yard work are all forms of physical activity. Include this type of activity in your daily routine.

Get Walking!

For most people walking is a good place to begin because it is easy and requires no special equipment other than a pair of good walking shoes or sneakers. If you choose to walk and have not exercised in a long time, you may need to begin by walking at a moderate pace. Walking about three times a week for a period of ten to fifteen minutes can help ease you into a routine. As you become stronger and gain more endurance, gradually increase your walking time by five minutes every one to two weeks, until you are able to walk for a full thirty minutes. Once you are comfortable walking for thirty minutes, increase your frequency to four or five times weekly, and gradually pick up the pace to a brisk walk. Brisk walking is considered an aerobic exercise, which means oxygen is used. Aerobic exercise increases your heart rate and burns calories. Walking in this manner is considered an effective type of exercise for weight loss. In addition to brisk walking, running, jogging, dancing, cycling, and swimming are examples of aerobic exercise. Generally, the more vigorous the aerobic exercise and the longer time you do it, the more benefits you will gain.

An excellent way to stay motivated and track your progress with walking is to use a pedometer. A *pedometer* is an inexpensive, small device that counts the number of steps you take in the course of the day. A pedometer is usually clipped to a belt or waistband, and if worn from the beginning to the end of your day, will count each step that you take. You can determine your daily step total by wearing the pedometer for three consecutive full days, then dividing the step total by three. Once you know the average steps you take per day, you can set small goals for yourself to increase the total number of steps you take every day.

QUESTION

What is the best time of day to exercise?
As long as you exercise, the time of day you actually do the exercise is the best time! Busy and demanding schedules often get in the way of good intentions. If your schedule is particularly demanding, try making an appointment on your schedule for your exercise time. Remember that any time spent exercising is better than no time!

To learn more about walking and using a pedometer, you may want to visit the site *www.shapeup.org/shape/steps.php*. The Shape Up America website can help you learn more about walking as a means to lose weight and improve fitness. The site provides encouragement and guidance for reaching 10,000 steps a day!

No Exercise = Little to No Results: It's a Must!

If you really want to stop pre-diabetes in its tracks, it is important to understand just how important it is to initiate a plan for physical activity. Many people just focus on changing their eating habits. While this is very important, the lack of exercise could prevent you from reaching your goals. Cutting down on food will not be enough to help you lose weight and maintain a lower weight. Physical activity is a key component to your pre-diabetes plan and must be included at whatever level you are able to accommodate. Exercise is often left out because of perceived barriers that keep someone from becoming more active. If you are someone who never seems able to find the time or energy for exercise, begin to take a serious look at what the barriers are. Once you identify what is getting in your way, plan strategies to help you go around those barriers. Keep your strategies simple and real. Writing down and implementing your strategy is a good way to help you make permanent changes.

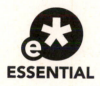

ESSENTIAL

Consistent exercise provides many rewards for everyone and especially for people with pre-diabetes. Preventing or delaying diabetes is at the top of the list, but you will also enjoy lower blood glucose and A1c levels, lower blood pressure, lower lipid levels, a more toned body, reduced stress, and better sleep!

Slow and Steady Wins the Race

Once you have had success with starting and maintaining your exercise, branch out and find new ways to get exercise and keep it interesting. Varying the routine helps to keep you from getting bored, and it challenges your body in different ways. An exercise plan of walking can be augmented by including strength training and stretching. Strength training helps to build muscle. Increasing muscle mass reduces insulin resistance and helps to lower blood glucose. Examples of strength training include lifting weights, push-ups, squats, lunges, and pull-ups. If you include strength training, be sure to allow at least forty-eight hours between sessions so your muscles are able to rest and recover. For most people, short strength training sessions two to three times weekly will provide added benefit. Stretching is another worthy addition to a well-rounded exercise plan because it helps to increase flexibility and prevent injury. Stretch slowly, without bouncing, and only stretch as far as you can without causing any pain. A few minutes of stretching at the beginning and end of an exercise session can make exercise easier and reduce the possibility of injury.

Your exercise program should be one that you can maintain for life. Make sensible decisions about what you can and will change to increase your activity level. You may realize some the benefits of exercise early on, but long-lasting results come about with consistency. Think of your exercise program as a work in progress which you are constantly improving and finding new ways to derive health benefits and enjoyment from. Slow, steady progress will help you achieve your goals, and you will realize how worthwhile your efforts have been.

CHAPTER 5

What Can I Eat?

You may think that having pre-diabetes means you will have to give up everything you like to eat, especially carbohydrates. Nothing could be further from the truth! With the help and advice from a registered dietitian, you can adapt healthy eating habits that fit into your lifestyle. Realize that you won't be able to change your eating habits overnight. It is much easier to adopt the approach of taking small steps every day. Over time, you can make significant changes toward improving your health and reaching near-normal blood glucose levels consistently.

Keep It Simple to Start

Think of changes in your eating habits as goals rather than inflexible rules and regulations. Start by making an honest review of your current eating habits and list the things you would like to change or improve. If you brainstorm a bit, you will be able to come up with quite a few positive changes that you could make. Decide exactly what you need to do in order to bring about change, and then select one or two changes to work on at a time. Here are a few ideas to help you start this process:

- Eat meals at regular intervals—resolve not to skip meals or go for long periods of time without eating.
- Include nutritious snacks in your daily eating plan—fruits and vegetables are good choices.
- Experiment with whole grains, vegetables, or fruits you have never tried before—check out the produce or whole foods section of your grocery store to see what's new.
- Start reducing your portion sizes—cut back by 25–30 percent to get used to eating less.
- Drink plenty of water every day.

Once you've mastered a change, it's time to move on to something new. Some changes will be easy, and others will be difficult or take more time. Start by making easier changes first before tackling something that would be very difficult for you. This will help build your confidence.

A Quick Primer on Nutrition: Balance and Moderation Are Key

Everyone has the same nutritional needs regardless of whether or not they have pre-diabetes. You may be surprised to learn that your eating plan will have the same foods that everyone else eats (or *should* be eating!), and buying all sorts of specialty or diet foods is usually unnecessary. You may wish to use an artificial sweetener of your choice or certain sugar-free food items to add variety, however this is not essential. You will not have to prepare one meal for yourself and something different for the rest of your family. As you look over the recipes in this book, you may want to try a few specialty items, but the recipes in general use ingredients that everyone can eat. To put it simply, a meal plan for managing pre-diabetes is a plan that most people can follow for good health.

ESSENTIAL

Eating a balanced diet that includes foods from all of the essential food groups generally meets the nutrition needs of most adults. Some individuals have other health issues in addition to pre-diabetes, and this may affect specific nutritional requirements. Discuss all of your health issues with your doctor and registered dietitian to determine whether you should take vitamin and mineral supplements to help meet specific nutritional needs.

Carbohydrates and Pre-Diabetes: Facts You Should Know

Carbohydrates serve as the body's primary energy source. Simple carbohydrates include sugars, sweets, juices, and fruits. Complex carbohydrates include all types of grain products and starchy vegetables such as potatoes and corn. Recommendations for a healthy diet and pre-diabetes suggest that most carbohydrate come from the complex carbohydrates rather than simple sugars. Complex carbohydrates found in whole grain foods provide better nutritional value and are an important source of vitamins, minerals, and fiber. Fruit contains natural, simple sugars, and they are also sources of vitamins, minerals, and fiber. To get the most fiber from fruit choose fresh or frozen, unsweetened fruit instead of fruit juice.

Having pre-diabetes or diabetes does not mean you must cut out all carbohydrates from your diet. You will be happy to learn that there are many carbohydrate food choices that you can include in your plan! Choose carbohydrates that have good nutritional value and maintain an appropriate portion size.

Protein: Your Building Blocks to Good Health

Proteins are the building blocks of the body and are used for growth, building, and repair. Animal proteins such as meat, fish, eggs, and milk contain all nine essential amino acids. When all essential amino acids are present in food, it is called a *complete protein*.

Vegetable proteins are found in nuts, seeds, vegetables, whole grains, and legumes. All vegetable proteins, with the exception of soy, are considered incomplete proteins because one or more of the essential amino acids are missing. Even though a vegetable protein is considered incomplete, it is not considered less nutritious than a complete protein. Incomplete proteins simply need to be combined with other foods to provide the full compliment of the nine essential amino acids. For example, combining rice (a grain) with beans (a legume) provides all of the essential amino acids. Combining grains, beans, nuts, vegetables, or seeds in various ways can provide a complete protein.

QUESTION

What are whole grains?
The FDA has defined *whole grains* as "the intact, ground, cracked, or flaked fruit of the grains whose principal components—the starchy endosperm, germ and bran—are present in the same relative proportions as they exist in the intact grain." In other words, no part of the grain has been removed during processing and so you are getting all of the parts of a grain.

Fats: Polys, Monos, Saturated, an

All fats, regardless of the type, ha
Therefore, moderation of any fat is your
tains 9 calories.

Monounsaturated fat should make up
type of fat is found in certain plant foods
oil, and olive oil. Monounsaturated fat do
may actually help reduce blood cholester
in the diet.

Polyunsaturated fat should be used in
monounsaturated fat. This fat come mostly   ources such as
corn oil, sunflower oil, and some types of margarine.

Saturated fat should be used the least. This type of fat is typically found in foods made from animal sources such as meat, butter, cheese, or cream. Baked goods such as cakes or pastries may be high in saturated fat if lard, palm, or coconut oils are used. Excessive intake of saturated fat can increase blood cholesterol levels.

Trans fat is the result of a food manufacturing process called *hydrogenation*. This process converts a liquid vegetable oil to a solid fat to make shortenings and solid (stick) types of margarine.

Foods containing omega-3 fatty acids are encouraged. Omega-3 plays an important role in the maintenance of immune function, brain development, and reproduction. There is considerable evidence to suggest that omega-3 fatty acids can have a positive effect on certain conditions due to its anti-inflammatory properties. Omega-3 fatty acids are found in soy oil, green leafy vegetables, walnuts, flax seed, and most notably, oily fish such as salmon, sardines, and mackerel.

ALERT

Check food labels and ingredients to avoid trans fat as much as possible. This form of fat can raise LDL (bad) cholesterol and increase your risk for heart disease. Trans fat can be found in vegetable shortenings, solid margarines, certain crackers, cookies, and other foods made with partially hydrogenated oils.

Cholesterol

Cholesterol is a waxy substance found in all body cells. It is part of some hormones and essential for fat digestion. The liver manufactures much of the cholesterol our body needs, but cholesterol is also obtained from the foods we eat. Cholesterol is found in animal foods such as meat, eggs, butter, and whole dairy products. Too much cholesterol in the blood can increase one's risk for heart disease. People with pre-diabetes or diabetes have more risk for heart disease and should have their blood cholesterol checked routinely. Limit consumption of fatty meats, butter, and whole dairy foods such as whole milk or whole milk cheeses. Your doctor or registered dietitian may provide you with more specific recommendations for cholesterol control.

Sodium

Sodium is a mineral that does not affect blood sugar, but it can alter your blood pressure. Controlling blood pressure is yet another important aspect of managing pre-diabetes and preventing heart disease. The current recommended sodium intake for healthy adults states to consume no more than 2,300 mg of sodium per day. The Dietary Guidelines for Americans are currently under revision, and there are discussions to incrementally reduce the sodium intake recommendation from 2,300 mg to 1,500 mg daily, using stepwise approach. This will mean people with higher calorie needs will have a slightly higher sodium allowance compared to those with lower calorie requirements. Overall, the recommendation will be lower for everyone.

Tips for reducing sodium:

- Leave out or reduce the amount of salt in standard recipes by 25–50 percent.
- Use commercial herb blends (or make your own using the recipes in Chapter 17 of this book) to season food instead of using salt.
- Limit intake of highly processed foods such as boxed mixes, instant foods, or processed meats.
- Make more soups, stews, casseroles, or side dishes from scratch.
- Watch your use of the salt shaker when cooking or at the table.

About Carbs, Fiber, and Whole Grains

There are two types of fiber found in foods: soluble and insoluble. It's important to include foods containing both types of fiber in your daily eating plan.

Soluble fiber dissolves or swells when it's put into water. Soluble fiber helps keep blood sugar levels stable by slowing down the rate of glucose absorption into the bloodstream. Soluble fiber, when consumed in adequate amounts, can help lower blood cholesterol levels as well. Beans, fruit, barley, and oats are especially good sources of soluble fiber. Insoluble fiber does not dissolve in water. In the body, it is not readily broken down by bacteria in the intestinal tract and this type of fiber passes through the body.

Insoluble fiber is essential for preventing constipation and diverticulosis by helping to maintain regularity. Vegetables, whole-grain foods, and fruit are all good sources of insoluble fiber.

Getting More Fiber Every Day

Although all types of grains are sources of complex carbohydrates, those that have not been refined are better for you. Whole grains have more fiber and minerals. Whole grains have not had the bran layer and germ removed during the milling process therefore the fiber, as well as vitamins and minerals are preserved. In addition, fiber helps to slow down the absorption of glucose into the bloodstream, which is important in the management of blood glucose. Refined grains such as white flour or white rice have the bran and germ removed. Refined grains are much lower in fiber, and vitamins and minerals are also removed during this process. Refined grains must have certain vitamins and minerals added back into the product after processing. Adding back nutrients to a processed food is called *enrichment*. When a label lists enriched flour as an ingredient, odds are it has been refined and may not be very high in fiber. Eating refined grains instead of whole grains makes it difficult to achieve adequate amounts of fiber each day. Whenever you can, choose whole grains over refined grains. The recommendation for daily fiber intake is 25–30g per day, which is about twice the amount found in the typical American diet.

FACT

Words like *multigrain*, *seven-grain*, or *stone-ground* do not necessarily mean a product is whole grain. If a whole-grain ingredient is not listed as the first ingredient, the item may contain only a small portion of whole grains. One way to find a whole grain product is to look for the Whole Grains Council stamp of approval, which has two different logos used to label foods containing whole grains. The logo that reads "100% Whole Grain" indicates that the food has only whole grains and at least 16g per serving. The other label indicates only that a product contains whole grains.

Great Ways to Get More Whole Grains

The best way to get more whole grains in your meals is to substitute whole-grain foods for refined products. Here are some tips:

- When a recipe calls for white flour (all-purpose), experiment by replacing some of the flour with a whole-grain variety.
- Use a whole grain as a side dish or mix it with vegetables, lentils, or beans.
- Every week try one "new" grain that you have not used before. Quinoa, brown rice, bulgur, or kasha may be unfamiliar to you, but are as easy to prepare as white rice.
- Add whole grains to soups, salads, or casseroles instead of white rice or pasta.
- Try a cooked whole grain as a hot breakfast cereal.
- If you are not used to bran or other high fiber cereals, try mixing with equal amounts of your regular cereal.
- Switch to whole-grain crackers instead of saltines or other white-flour snack crackers.
- Use oatmeal in place of bread crumbs in items such as meatloaf or meatballs.
- Gradually start replacing the refined grains in your kitchen cabinets with whole-grain foods.

Gluten-Free Whole Grains

Consider adding gluten-free whole grains to your eating plan, even if you don't have celiac disease or a gluten/wheat intolerance. Many gluten-free whole grains are a wonderful source of fiber and essential nutrients. Gluten-free whole grains are available in their whole form or as flours. A few examples to consider include amaranth, buckwheat, teff, sorghum, quinoa, and montina (Indian rice grass).

CHAPTER 6

Translating Nutrition into Real Meals

Knowing about good nutrition or the types of foods that you should eat when you have pre-diabetes is not enough. Translating what you know into an actual plan with healthy meals is very important! In this chapter you will learn more about using nutrition information to make wiser food choices whether you are shopping for food, dining out, or preparing your own meals.

Reading Food Labels

The Nutrition Facts found on food labels contain plenty of information, but unless you understand how to read the labels, you may be presented with information that doesn't mean very much to you.

Understanding Terms on Labels

Serving Size: Each label must identify the size of a serving. The nutritional information listed on a label is based on one serving of the food. Note that the serving listed on a package may not be the same as the size of your serving.

Amount per Serving: Each package identifies the quantities of nutrients and food constituents from one serving. From this information, you can find the caloric value of the food, in addition to how much fat (saturated or trans fat), cholesterol, sodium, carbohydrates, and protein per serving.

Percent Daily Value: This indicates how much of a specific nutrient a serving of food contains in comparison to an average 2,000 calorie diet.

Ingredient List: A listing of the ingredients in a food in descending order of predominance and weight.

Compare Carbohydrate Grams to Grams of Sugar

There are several parts to the carbohydrate section of the nutrition label. *Total Carbohydrates* represent the amount of carbohydrate grams found in a food. If the amount of carbohydrate grams is very high, you may decide whether or not it will fit into your eating plan. Beneath the Total Carbohydrates line are other listings: Fiber, Sugars, and sometimes, Sugar Alcohols. These values are part of Total Carbohydrate.

ESSENTIAL

By comparing the calories from fat to the total calories in a food, you can identify foods that have lots of hidden fat. A typical hot dog has 110 total calories and 90 calories from fat. This means that 82 percent of the calories in the hot dog come from fat! Making this determination before buying a food can help you make much healthier choices. Look for foods that have 30 percent or less of the calories from fat.

When you find the grams of Sugars in a product, be sure to compare it to the grams of Total Carbohydrate. For example, if a cup of cereal has 32g Total Carbohydrate and 16g of Sugars, that means 50 percent of the carbohydrate in the cereal comes from Sugars. Try to choose foods with 25 percent or less grams of Sugars, so that you make food choices with lower amounts of sugars. Use this guideline only for food items where sugar is added to the foods. Items such as milk, yogurt, or fruit have naturally occurring sugar and do not fall into this category unless sugar has been added to the product.

Fiber grams are also part of Total Carbohydrate. Choose higher fiber foods by selecting those that contain 4 or more grams of fiber per serving.

The Glycemic Index

The *glycemic index* (GI) measures how a food with carbohydrate raises blood glucose. Foods are ranked on a scale from 0–100, based on a comparison to a reference food. Using the GI involves choosing foods that have a low or medium GI more often, and limiting foods known to have a high GI. Examples of carbohydrate foods with a low GI include dried beans and legumes, non-starchy vegetables, most whole fruits, and many whole-grain breads and cereals. Foods that do not contain carbohydrates (such as meats and fats) do not have a GI. Foods that are good sources of fiber tend to have a lower GI. In general, the less processed a food is, the lower the GI. The GI of a food can be affected by its degree of ripeness, the amount and type of processing a food has sustained, or the method in which a food has been cooked. For example, a very ripe piece of fruit will have a higher GI than one that is not as ripe. Pasta that is cooked al dente has a lower GI than soft cooked pasta.

When it comes to meal planning for pre-diabetes or diabetes, there is no right way that works for everyone. The American Diabetes Association recommends using methods such as carbohydrate counting or food exchanges as the key means for monitoring total carbohydrate intake. The use of low GI as a secondary method may provide a modest additional benefit for glycemic control. If you choose to use the GI as a meal-planning tool, keep in mind the total amount of carbohydrate that you eat is still the most important factor. For more information about the glycemic index go to: *www .joslin.org* or *www.mendosa.com/gilists.htm*.

Grocery Lists and Your Kitchen Makeover

Having a plan and the right foods on hand is the best way to keep you eating healthier. If you don't have a good plan and leave things up to chance, you could make poor food choices. Grabbing fast-food or take-out meals at the last minute usually means you will be eating fewer vegetables, fresh fruit, or whole-grain foods. At the same time, you will be consuming plenty of calories, fat, and refined or highly processed foods.

Set aside some time each week to plan your meals. If you work or have a very busy schedule, a good time to plan or shop may be your day off or a quiet time of the day. A little bit of time invested in meal planning saves overall time and money throughout the week.

Keep a weekly shopping list visible and handy; when you think of food items you need, write them on your list. Each time you plan, consider what meals and snacks you will need for the coming week. As you develop a shopping list, take stock of the types of foods you have in your kitchen cabinets, refrigerator, and freezer, then decide what type of items need to be added to your grocery list.

Having plenty of healthy food choices available all of the time helps you avoid the pitfalls of eating too many empty-calorie foods that get in the way of weight loss or managing your diabetes.

TWENTY FOODS TO ALWAYS HAVE ON HAND
1. Vegetables: Any fresh, frozen, or reduced sodium canned
2. Fruits: Any fresh, frozen (unsweetened), or canned (juice or water-packed)
3. Whole-grain bread
4. High-fiber (low-sugar) cereals with 4g or more fiber per serving
5. Canned beans, dry beans, or lentils: Any variety
6. Boneless, skinless chicken or turkey breast
7. Egg substitutes or egg whites
8. Tuna or salmon canned in water
9. Low-fat cheese or cheese sticks—choose 1–1½ %-fat varieties
10. Nonstick cooking spray
11. Dried herbs and spices: Any single varieties or mixes made without the addition of salt
12. Dry roasted or raw nuts: walnuts and almonds are good choices

13. Non-caloric sweetener
14. Reduced-fat mayonnaise or salad dressing
15. Low-sodium chicken, vegetable, or beef broth
16. Leafy lettuce varieties or bagged salad mixes using leafy varieties
17. One or more whole grains: quinoa, amaranth, barley, bulgur, kasha, brown rice, or whole-grain pasta
18. Canned tomatoes or stewed canned tomatoes
19. Fat-free yogurt: plain, vanilla, or fruit flavored, artificially sweetened
20. Whole-grain crackers

When you go shopping, let your shopping list guide you and stick to your list as much as possible. The healthiest foods are found around the perimeter of the store, and everything else is found in the aisles. Spend most of your time shopping around the perimeter.

Make Over Your Food Supply

Making over your kitchen food supply does not have to be extreme, costly or stressful. You can gradually makeover your kitchen cupboards by phasing out foods of lesser nutritional quality with newer ones that have more health benefits or lower calories. As you run out of items that you already have, replace the item with something new.

▼ **SUGGESTIONS FOR SWITCHING TO HEALTHIER FOODS**

Instead of:	Replace it with:
Garlic or Onion Salt	Fresh Garlic or Onion
Fruit Juices	Fresh Fruit
All-Purpose Flour	Whole-Wheat or Rye Flour
Vegetable Oil	Olive or Canola Oil
Sour Cream	Plain Low-Fat Yogurt
Buttery Snack Crackers	Whole-Grain Crackers
Cookies	Graham Crackers
Potato Chips	Popcorn (make your own)
Half Gallon of Ice Cream	Single-Serving, Reduced-Calorie Ice Cream
Bacon	Thin-Sliced, Low-Fat Ham

Tips for Dining Out

For many Americans, work schedules and busy lifestyles have made dining out a common and frequent occurrence. Eating out can present lots of challenges when your goals are to maintain a healthy eating plan and lose weight. As with other aspects of managing your health, it's important to plan and learn about strategies for healthier eating when you go out to eat. Many people consider restaurant meals a special occasion and this can mean a time to splurge on desserts or rich foods. If you dine out frequently, viewing meals out as special occasions will sabotage your efforts to eat healthier. Take a closer look at how often you dine out, the type of food you order, and how much food you eat. Some of the pitfalls with eating out include frequent visits to fast-food restaurants or simply eating out often because you do not keep enough healthy foods available at home.

Avoiding Hidden Fats

It's no secret that many restaurant foods include plenty of oils, butter, cream, sauces, or cheeses in their preparation. Fats contribute to the flavor and taste of food, but that's where lots of extra calories come in. Foods prepared with large amounts of fat will have a higher caloric content. Healthy salad greens, for example, can end up being very high in calories if laden with large amounts of salad dressing and toppings.

The Portion Problem

One of the biggest challenges with eating out is coping with the large portions served. Unfortunately getting more food is considered a greater value, as evidenced by value meals, all-you-can-eat, or dollar incentives for extra-large options. When you eat out, be prepared to receive large portions, and have a strategy of your own to deal with this situation. If you know too much food is served at a particular restaurant, try ordering from the appetizer, soup, or salad section of the menu. Ask for a container when your meal is served and put ⅓ to ½ of the meal in the container *before* you start eating. You'll eat much less food that way, and have an extra meal to take home and eat later.

The best restaurant menu picks include:

- Dishes prepared with tomato sauces rather than cream sauces
- Grilled, poached, or broiled fish or poultry dishes
- Grilled or broiled meats served without gravies or sauces
- Vegetables that have been steamed or lightly sautéed
- Broth-based soups instead of cream soups
- Salads with dressing on the side and minus the extras such as cheese and croutons

ALERT

Restaurant meals can sound healthy, but be on the lookout for extra fats that may be added to the food. Cream sauces, melted cheese, sour cream, or stir frying can add extra calories. A mere teaspoon of oil or butter provides 45–50 calories. You can take some of the guesswork out of choosing from a menu when you ask how a dish is prepared. Having this information can help you decide whether it fits into your healthy eating plan.

What about Alcohol?

When it comes to alcohol and your health, the optimal word is always *moderation*. Consider the facts about alcohol and decide whether including alcohol on a moderate basis fits into your pre-diabetes management plan. Alcohol does not provide any essential nutrients, but it is a source of calories. If you drink and are having difficulty losing weight, do not overlook the calories that alcohol adds to your overall intake. Alcohol can impact blood lipid levels and elevate triglycerides. Both of these health issues may already be a source of concern for you.

It is perfectly okay to add a small amount of alcohol in certain recipes. A bit of wine or flavored liqueur can enhance the flavor of the food, and can be incorporated as a low-fat cooking ingredient or marinade. When cooked, the alcohol content diminishes, but the flavor remains.

What does alcohol in moderation mean?
Moderation is considered to be two drinks a day for men and one drink a day for women. One drink is a 12-ounce beer, 5 ounce glass of wine, or 1½ ounces of distilled spirits. Beverages with mixers (sodas, juices, etc.) have more carbohydrates. If you use mixers, lower the calories and carbohydrates by using club soda, mineral water, diet soda, or diet tonic water in the drink.

Making Recipe Adjustments for Your New Cooking Style

Your favorite recipes can be adjusted to lower fat, salt, or sugar content, yet still maintain good taste. Recipes that are cooked stove-top rather than baked can often turn out quite well with a simple reduction in sugar, salt, or fat. It is possible to substitute low-fat or low-sodium ingredients in certain recipes. As an example, using 1% milk instead of whole milk in a pudding recipe lowers fat and calories without significantly altering the taste.

Can sugar be eliminated from my favorite cake and cookie recipes?
Completely eliminating sugar from baked desserts can be tricky. Although sugar is an empty-calorie food, it does serve as an important ingredient in certain baked foods by enhancing the flavor, texture, and appearance of the end product. When sugar is reduced or replaced with an artificial sweetener in a cake or cookie recipe, the result can be very different and not what you were hoping for. The baked good can be denser, lack a golden brown color, or have a flavor unlike the original recipe.

Some of the recipes found in this cookbook may contain ingredients such as butter or salt in small amounts. These ingredients are usually part of a recipe because they improve the flavor of a food or aid in the baking process. When baking bread, cookies, or cakes, salt is usually required in the leavening process and should not be eliminated. If you must eliminate all butter from your diet most recipes can use soft spread margarines or vegetable oil as a substitute. You and your dietitian can decide whether it is appropriate to include these ingredients in small quantities or make a substitution.

The recipes for baked desserts found in this cookbook have different methods for addressing sugar. Some recipes will simply have a reduction in the total amount of sugar used. There are other recipes that use a different type of sugar that has caloric value, such as honey or maple syrup. When these are used in the place of sugar, a lesser quantity is used; therefore the end product is lower in sugar, but not sugar-free. Lastly, some recipes have a combination of an artificial sweetener with a very small amount of regular sugar. As you work with these or with your own recipes, you will learn how to adjust ingredients to get good results.

Tips for Replacing or Reducing Sugar and Fat

Try reducing a standard recipe's sugar content by 25–50 percent. It's usually best to start with a smaller reduction (25 percent) and gradually decrease the amount of sugar each time the product is made. Be sure to note whether the properties of the food have any significant or undesirable changes, then adjust as needed.

Use puréed, unsweetened fruit or fruit juices to replace some or all of the sugar in a recipe.

Honey or maple syrup are sugars and will affect blood sugar, however, either can add sweetness to a food. Carbohydrate and calories can be reduced in a recipe if you use a smaller amount of these sugars in a recipe.

Many recipes can withstand up to a 50 percent reduction in fat. To replace fat, but not volume, try using plain yogurt, applesauce, mashed ripe banana, or other puréed fruit for half of the oil or shortening called for in a recipe. If the product requires sweetness in addition to volume, applesauce or mashed ripe banana make good options.

Using Sugar Substitutes

Sugar substitutes are never mandatory for when you have pre-diabetes, but they can offer options to those who wish to use them. Using a sugar substitute in a recipe can slash sugar content and a significant amount of calories. When using sugar substitutes in baking, keep in mind that sweetness is being added to the food, but other traits unique to a baked product (volume, texture, golden-brown color) may be altered.

The sweeteners listed below are all approved by the FDA. They vary in taste, uses, and suitability for cooking or baking. You will need to do a taste test on your own to decide which ones are best for you.

▼ **SUGAR SUBSTITUTES**

Sweetener	Brand Name	Notes
Saccharin	Sweet N'Low® or Sugar Twin®	Saccharin can leave a bitter aftertaste, and may need to be combined with other sweeteners to improve taste when used in cooking. 24 packets replaces 1 cup of sugar.
Aspartame	Equal® or NutraSweet®	High temperatures diminish sweetness, making this product less suitable for baking. Aspartame contains phenylalanine, which can be harmful to people with the rare disease Phenylketonuria (PKU) and it must be avoided by them.
Sucralose	Splenda®	There are several baking products using sucralose, including a granular version that measures cup for cup with sugar. There are also half sugar and brown sugar blends, which contain sugar, so adjust accordingly.
Stevia	Truvia®, PureVia®	Look for brands of stevia that use a purified portion of the stevia leaf known as *rebaudioside A*. Sugar to stevia ratios vary with each brand, so follow recommendations by the manufacturer if using in cooking or baking.

Cooking Styles

There are many ways to prepare foods that not only preserve nutrients and good taste, but also minimize the use of sugar, salt, and fat. A little creativity with spices, herbs, or combining foods together in unconventional ways makes food more flavorful without the addition of extra fat, sodium, or calories. Stir frying, broiling, and slow cooking are examples of techniques that are time saving and result in more healthful food.

The principle of stir frying uses a very small amount of oil and cooks foods quickly at a high heat. It allows you to combine several foods together for a quick and healthy meal. Foods that work well using the stir fry method include vegetables, poultry, meats, fish, and cooked grains. When stir frying, choose oil with a high smoke point such as canola or peanut oil to allow for a high cooking temperature. Remember to use as little oil as possible; usually 1–2 teaspoons will do. Stir fried foods from a restaurant menu may be very different from a home prepared version. Before selecting a restaurant stir fried dish, ask how the food is prepared and how much oil is being used.

Broiling or grilling involves cooking foods on a rack to allow fats to drip to a pan or flame below. Most meats, poultry, or fish can be grilled or broiled. Broiling instead of cooking in oil can reduce fat and calories. When using an outdoor grill, use aluminum foil to minimize the direct contact of food with the flame, and be sure to prevent foods from charring or over browning.

Slow cookers are often overlooked, but can be very helpful in the preparation of healthy meals. They are extremely easy to use and can save a lot of time in the kitchen. Foods are placed in the slow cooker early in the day and allowed to cook at a low temperature for several hours or more. Meals made in a slow cooker do not require the addition of fats, and the slow cooking helps tenderize tougher cuts of meat. Soups, sauces, and stews are just a few examples of the items you can cook in a slow cooker.

You can start putting your pre-diabetes plan into action by cooking more at home and using healthier styles of cooking.

Breakfast Fare

Egg White Pancakes

NUTRITIONAL ANALYSIS (per serving):

Calories: 197 Protein: 13g Carbohydrates: 31g Fat: 3g Saturated Fat: 1g Cholesterol: 0mg
Sodium: 120mg Fiber: 4g PCF Ratio: 27-61-12 Exchange Approx.: 1 Free Sweet, 1 Lean Meat, 1½ Breads

INGREDIENTS | SERVES 2

4 egg whites

½ cup oatmeal

4 teaspoons reduced-calorie or low-sugar strawberry jam

1 teaspoon powdered sugar

Creative Toppings

Experiment with toast and pancake toppings. Try a tablespoon of raisins, almonds, apples, bananas, berries, nut butters (limit these to 1 teaspoon per serving), peanuts, pears, walnuts, or wheat germ.

1. Put all ingredients in blender; process until smooth.

2. Preheat nonstick pan treated with cooking spray over medium heat. Pour half of mixture into pan; cook for 4–5 minutes.

3. Flip pancake and cook until inside is cooked. Repeat using remaining batter for second pancake. Dust each pancake with powdered sugar, if using.

Buckwheat Pancakes

NUTRITIONAL ANALYSIS (per serving):

Calories: 220   Protein: 11g   Carbohydrates: 44g   Fat: 1g   Saturated Fat: 0g   Cholesterol: 1mg
Sodium: 200mg   Fiber: 5g   PCF Ratio: 76-19-5   Exchange Approx.: 2 Starches, ½ Skim Milk, ½ Fruit

INGREDIENTS | SERVES 2

1 cup whole-wheat flour
½ cup buckwheat flour
1½ teaspoons baking powder
2 egg whites
¼ cup apple juice concentrate
1¼ to 1½ cups skim milk

1. Sift flours and baking powder together. Combine egg whites, apple juice concentrate, and 1¼ cups milk. Add milk mixture to dry ingredients; mix well, but do not over-mix. Add remaining milk if necessary to reach desired consistency.

2. Cook pancakes in nonstick skillet or on griddle treated with nonstick spray over medium heat.

Berry Puff Pancakes

NUTRITIONAL ANALYSIS (per serving):

Calories: 110   Protein: 5g   Carbohydrates: 37g   Fat: 2g   Saturated Fat: 1g   Cholesterol: 71mg
Sodium: 89mg   Fiber: 3g   PCF Ratio: 65-18-17   Exchange Approx.: 1 Starch, ½ Fruit

INGREDIENTS | SERVES 6

2 large whole eggs
1 large egg white
½ cup skim milk
½ cup all-purpose flour
1 tablespoon granulated sugar
⅛ teaspoon sea salt
2 cups of fresh berries such as raspberries, blackberries, boysenberries, blueberries, strawberries, or a combination
1 tablespoon powdered sugar

Syrup Substitutes

Spreading 2 teaspoons of your favorite Smucker's Low-Sugar jam or jelly on a waffle or pancake not only gives you a sweet topping, it can be one of your Free Exchange List choices for the day.

1. Preheat oven to 450°F. Treat 10" ovenproof skillet or deep pie pan with nonstick spray. Once oven is heated, place pan in oven for a few minutes to get hot.

2. Add eggs and egg white to medium bowl; beat until mixed. Whisk in milk. Slowly whisk in flour, sugar, and salt.

3. Remove preheated pan from oven; pour batter into it. Bake for 15 minutes; reduce heat to 350°F and bake for an additional 10 minutes, or until batter is puffed and brown. Remove from oven and slide onto serving plate. Cover with fruit and sift powdered sugar over top. Cut into 6 equal wedges and serve.

Buttermilk Pancakes

NUTRITIONAL ANALYSIS (per serving):

Calories: 143   Protein: 6g   Carbohydrates: 26g   Fat: 2g   Saturated Fat: 1g   Cholesterol: 49mg
Sodium: 111mg   Fiber: 1g   PCF Ratio: 16-74-10   Exchange Approx.: 1½ Starches

INGREDIENTS | SERVES 2

1 cup all-purpose flour

2 tablespoons nonfat buttermilk powder

¼ teaspoon baking soda

½ teaspoon low-salt baking powder

1 cup water

1. Blend together all ingredients, adding more water if necessary to get batter consistency desired.

2. Pour ¼ of batter into nonstick skillet or skillet treated with nonstick cooking spray. Cook over medium heat until bubbles appear on top half of pancake. Flip and continue cooking until center of pancake is done. Repeat process with remaining batter.

Nut Butter Batter

For a change of pace, try adding 1 Exchange amount per serving of nut butter to pancake batter and use jelly or jam instead of syrup.

Sweet Potato Pancakes

NUTRITIONAL ANALYSIS (per serving):

Calories: 168   Protein: 6g   Carbohydrates: 25.87g   Fat: 7g   Saturated Fat: 1g   Cholesterol: 0mg
Sodium: 139mg   Fiber: 3g   PCF Ratio: 13-49-37   Exchange Approx.: 1 Starch, 1½ Fats

INGREDIENTS | SERVES 4

1½ cups sweet potatoes, cooked
¼ cup onions, grated
1 egg
3 tablespoons whole-wheat pastry flour
½ teaspoon cinnamon
½ teaspoon baking powder
½ cup egg whites
2 tablespoons canola oil

1. Scrub 2 medium sweet potatoes; pierce skins with fork and microwave on high for 4–5 minutes. When sweet potatoes have cooled enough to handle, scoop sweet potato out of skins; lightly mash with fork.

2. In medium bowl, mix together sweet potatoes, grated onion, and egg. Add in flour, cinnamon, and baking powder.

3. In separate small bowl, beat egg whites until rounded peaks are formed. Gently fold egg whites into potato mixture.

4. Heat oil in skillet (nonstick preferably) until hot. Spoon batter onto skillet to form pancakes approximately 4" in diameter. Brown on both sides.

5. Serve hot with unsweetened applesauce.

Country-Style Omelet

NUTRITIONAL ANALYSIS (per serving):

Calories: 253   Protein: 17g   Carbohydrates: 7g   Fat: 17g   Saturated Fat: 5g   Cholesterol: 493mg
Sodium: 221mg   Fiber: 2g   PCF Ratio: 27-12-61   Exchange Approx.: 1 Vegetable, 2 Medium-Fat Meats, 3 Fats

INGREDIENTS | SERVES 2

2 teaspoons olive oil

1 cup zucchini, diced

¼ cup red pepper, diced

1 cup plum tomatoes, skinned and cubed

⅛ teaspoon pepper

4 eggs

1 tablespoon Parmesan cheese

1 teaspoon fresh basil, minced

1. Heat oil in nonstick skillet. Add zucchini and red pepper; sauté for 5 minutes.

2. Add tomatoes and pepper; cook uncovered for another 10 minutes, allowing fluid from tomatoes to cook down.

3. In small bowl, whisk together eggs, Parmesan cheese, and fresh basil; pour over vegetables in skillet.

4. Cook over low heat until browned, approximately 10 minutes on each side.

Fruit Smoothie

NUTRITIONAL ANALYSIS (per serving):

The Nutritional Analysis and Fruit Exchange for this recipe will depend on your choice of fruit. Otherwise, allow ½ Skim Milk Exchange and ½ Misc. Food Exchange. The wheat germ adds fiber, but at less than 20 calories a serving, it can count as 1 Free Exchange.

INGREDIENTS | SERVES 1

1 cup skim milk
2 Exchange servings of any diced fruit
1 tablespoon honey
4 teaspoons toasted wheat germ
6 large ice cubes

Put all ingredients into blender or food processor; process until thick and smooth.

Batch 'Em

Make large batches of smoothies so you can keep single servings in the freezer. Get out a serving as you begin to get ready for your day. This should give the smoothie time to thaw enough for you to stir it when you're ready to have breakfast.

Yogurt Fruit Smoothie

NUTRITIONAL ANALYSIS (per serving):

Calories: 149   Protein: 10g   Carbohydrates: 26g   Fat: 1g   Saturated Fat: 0g   Cholesterol: 2mg
Sodium: 96mg   Fiber: 2g   PCF Ratio: 25-67-8   Exchange Approx.: 1 Milk, 1 Fruit

INGREDIENTS | SERVES 2

1 cup plain low-fat yogurt
½ cup sliced strawberries
½ cup orange juice
½ cup nectarines, peeled and sliced
2 tablespoons ground flax seed

Put all ingredients in blender; process until smooth.

Variations and Combos

You can vary this smoothie by substituting other fruits of your choice. Good combinations are strawberry and banana, strawberry and kiwi, or banana and peach. Keep portions of each fruit to no more than ½ cup.

Tofu Smoothie

NUTRITIONAL ANALYSIS (per serving):

Calories: 289 Protein: 20g Carbohydrates: 35g Fat: 11g Saturated Fat: 2g Cholesterol: 0mg
Sodium: 19mg Fiber: 8g PCF Ratio: 25-44-31 Exchange Approx.: 1 Meat Substitute, 2 Fruits

INGREDIENTS | SERVES 1

1⅓ cups frozen unsweetened strawberries

½ banana

½ cup (4 ounces) silken tofu

In food processor or blender, process all ingredients until smooth. Add a little chilled water for thinner smoothies if desired.

Overnight Oatmeal

NUTRITIONAL ANALYSIS (per serving):

Calories: 221   Protein: 9g   Carbohydrates: 42g   Fat: 3g   Saturated Fat: 1g   Cholesterol: 1mg
Sodium: 25mg   Fiber: 6g   PCF Ratio: 15-73-11   Exchange Approx.: 1 Fruit, 1 Starch, ½ Skim Milk

INGREDIENTS | SERVES 4

1 cup steel-cut oats

14 dried apricot halves

1 dried fig

2 tablespoons golden raisins

4 cups water

½ cup Mock Cream (Chapter 16)

Add all ingredients to slow cooker with a ceramic interior; set to low heat. Cover and cook overnight (8–9 hours).

Another Overnight Method

For another way to cook steel-cut oats, place 1 cup steel cut oats, 4 cups water, and dried fruit in medium saucepan; bring to a quick boil. Turn off the heat and cover saucepan. When cooled, place in covered container and refrigerate overnight. In morning, the oatmeal will have absorbed all of the water. Scoop 1 portion of the oatmeal into a bowl; microwave on high for 1 ½ to 2 minutes. Add milk and serve. Heat up refrigerated leftover portions as needed; use within 3 days.

Egg Clouds on Toast

NUTRITIONAL ANALYSIS (per serving):

Calories: 57   Protein: 4g   Carbohydrates: 9g   Fat: 1g   Saturated Fat: 0g   Cholesterol: 0mg
Sodium: 101mg   Fiber: 0g   PCF Ratio: 30-63-7   Exchange Approx.: ½ Very-Lean Fat Meat, ½ Starch

INGREDIENTS | SERVES 1

2 egg whites

½ teaspoon sugar

1 cup water

1 tablespoon frozen apple juice concentrate

1 slice reduced-calorie oat-bran bread, lightly toasted

Tip

Additional serving suggestions: Spread 1 teaspoon of low-sugar or all-fruit spread on toast (½ Fruit Exchange) before ladling on the "clouds." For cinnamon French-style toast, sprinkle ¼ teaspoon cinnamon and ½ teaspoon powdered sugar (less than 10 calories) over top of the clouds.

1. In copper bowl, beat egg whites until thickened. Add sugar; continue to beat until stiff peaks form.

2. In small saucepan, heat water and apple juice over medium heat until it just begins to boil; reduce heat and allow mixture to simmer. Drop egg whites by teaspoonful into simmering water. Simmer for 3 minutes; turn over and simmer for an additional 3 minutes.

3. Ladle "clouds" over bread and serve immediately.

Quinoa Berry Breakfast

NUTRITIONAL ANALYSIS (per serving):

Calories: 228   Protein: 7g   Carbohydrates: 41g   Fat: 5g   Saturated Fat: 0g   Cholesterol: 0mg
Sodium: 2mg   Fiber: 5g   PCF Ratio: 12-69-19   Exchange Approx.: 2 Starches, 1 Fruit, 1 Very-Lean Meat, 4 Fats

INGREDIENTS | SERVES 4

1 cup quinoa
2 cups water
¼ cup walnuts
1 teaspoon cinnamon
2 cups berries

1. Rinse quinoa in fine-mesh sieve before cooking. Place quinoa, water, walnuts, and cinnamon in 1½ quart saucepan; bring to a boil. Reduce heat to low; cover and cook for 15 minutes, or until all water has been absorbed.

2. Add berries and serve with milk, soy milk, or sweetener if desired.

Single Serving Quick Tip

Use this basic recipe to make 4 servings at once. Refrigerated any leftover portions; microwave 1 to 1½ minutes on high for single portions as needed. Use cooked quinoa within 3 days. Try other berries, nuts, or spices such as ginger or nutmeg to vary this nutritious breakfast cereal.

CHAPTER 8

Soups

Lentil Soup with Herbs and Lemon

NUTRITIONAL ANALYSIS (per serving):

Calories: 214   Protein: 15g   Carbohydrates: 34g   Fat: 3g   Saturated Fat: 1g   Cholesterol: 0mg   Sodium: 353mg
Fiber: 16g   PCF Ratio: 27-61-12   Exchange Approx.: 1 Lean Meat, 2 Starches, 1 Vegetable

INGREDIENTS | SERVES 4

1 cup lentils, soaked overnight in 1 cup water

6 cups low-fat, reduced-sodium chicken broth

1 carrot, sliced

1 stalk celery, sliced

1 yellow onion, thinly sliced

2 teaspoons olive oil

1 tablespoon dried tarragon

½ teaspoon dried oregano

Sea salt and black pepper, to taste (optional)

1 tablespoon lemon juice

4 thin slices of lemon

1. Drain and rinse lentils. Add lentils and broth to pot over medium heat; bring to a boil. Reduce heat and simmer until tender, approximately 15 minutes. (If you did not presoak the lentils, increase cooking time by about 15 more minutes.)

2. While lentils are cooking, sauté carrot, celery, and onion in oil for 8 minutes, or until onion is golden brown. Remove from heat and set aside.

3. When lentils are tender, add vegetables, tarragon, oregano, and salt and pepper, if using; cook for 2 minutes. Stir in lemon juice. Ladle into 4 serving bowls; garnish with lemon slices.

Believe It or Not!

Put a fork at the bottom of the pan when you cook a pot of beans. The beans will cook in half the time.

Vegetable and Bean Chili

NUTRITIONAL ANALYSIS (per serving):

Calories: 205   Protein: 12g   Carbohydrates: 35g   Fat: 3g   Saturated Fat: 1g   Cholesterol: 0mg
Sodium: 156mg   Fiber: 13g   PCF Ratio: 22-65-13   Exchange Approx.: 1 Lean Meat, 2 Starches, 1 Vegetable

INGREDIENTS | SERVES 8

4 teaspoons olive oil

2 cups cooking onions, chopped

½ cup green bell pepper, chopped

3 cloves garlic, chopped

1 small jalapeño pepper, finely chopped (include the seeds if you like the chili extra hot)

1 tablespoon chili powder

1 teaspoon ground cumin

1 (28-ounce) can unsalted tomatoes, chopped and undrained

2 zucchinis, peeled and chopped

2 (15-ounce) cans unsalted kidney beans, rinsed

1 tablespoon chopped semisweet chocolate

3 tablespoons chopped fresh cilantro

1. Heat heavy pot over moderately high heat. Add olive oil, onions, bell pepper, garlic, and jalapeño; sauté until vegetables are softened, about 5 minutes. Add chili powder and cumin; sauté for 1 minute, stirring frequently to mix well.

2. Add tomatoes with juice and zucchini; bring to a boil. Lower heat and simmer, partially covered, for 15 minutes, stirring occasionally.

3. Stir in beans and chocolate; simmer, stirring occasionally, for additional 5 minutes, or until beans are heated through and chocolate is melted. Stir in cilantro, and serve.

Tomato-Vegetable Soup

NUTRITIONAL ANALYSIS (per serving):

Calories: 158   Protein: 5g   Carbohydrates: 31g   Fat: 3g   Saturated Fat: 1g   Cholesterol: 0mg
Sodium: 349mg   Fiber: 5g   PCF Ratio: 12-72-16   Exchange Approx.: 1½ Starches, 1 Vegetable

INGREDIENTS | SERVES 6

1 tablespoon olive oil

2 teaspoons minced garlic

⅔ teaspoon cumin

2 carrots, chopped

2 stalks celery, diced

1 medium onion, chopped

⅔ cup unsalted tomato paste

½ teaspoon red pepper flakes

2 cups canned unsalted peeled tomatoes, with juice

⅔ teaspoon chopped fresh oregano

3 cups low-fat, reduced-sodium chicken broth

3 cups fat-free beef broth

2 cups diced potatoes

2 cups shredded cabbage

½ cup green beans

½ cup fresh or frozen corn kernels

½ teaspoon freshly cracked black pepper

¼ cup lime juice or balsamic vinegar

1. Heat olive oil in large stockpot; sauté garlic, cumin, carrot, and celery 1 minute. Add onion; cook until transparent.

2. Stir in tomato paste; sauté until it begins to brown.

3. Add remaining ingredients except for lime juice or vinegar. Bring to a boil; reduce heat and simmer for 20–30 minutes, adding additional broth or water if needed. Just before serving, add lime juice or balsamic vinegar.

Easy Measures

Consider freezing broth in an ice cube tray. Most ice cube tray sections hold ⅛ cup (2 tablespoons) of liquid. Once broth is frozen, you can transfer cubes to freezer bag or container. This makes it easy to measure out the amount you need for recipes.

Minestrone Soup Genoese Style

NUTRITIONAL ANALYSIS (per serving):

Calories: 201 Protein: 9g Carbohydrates: 29g Fat: 6g Saturated Fat: 2g Cholesterol: 5mg
Sodium: 271mg Fiber: 6g PCF Ratio: 17-56-27 Exchange Approx.: 1½ Starches, 1 Vegetable, 1 Fat

INGREDIENTS | SERVES 6

4 cloves garlic, minced
2 tablespoons basil, chopped
¼ teaspoon salt
2 tablespoons olive oil
1 ounce Romano cheese
2 cups cabbage, shredded
1 cup zucchini, diced
1 cup green beans, cut into 1" pieces
1 cup potatoes, peeled and chopped
2 cups navy beans, cooked
½ cup celery, chopped
¼ cup peas, fresh or frozen
1 tablespoon tomato paste
3 cups water
Salt and pepper, to taste

1. Combine garlic, basil, and salt. Add olive oil and Romano cheese; mix well into a paste and set aside. (Using a mortar and pestle works very well.)

2. Combine cabbage, zucchini, green beans, potatoes, cooked navy beans, celery, peas, tomato paste, and water in a 4–6 quart soup pot.

3. Bring to a boil; reduce heat and simmer for 45–60 minutes, or until tender.

4. Mix garlic paste into soup; simmer an additional 5 minutes. Serve.

Tip

Make extra garlic paste (using first 5 ingredients and step 1) and keep refrigerated. You'll have instant garlic-cheese flavor on hand for soups, sauces, garlic bread, and pasta dishes. Garlic paste keeps in the refrigerator for up to 2 weeks.

Broccoli and Whole-Grain Pasta Soup

NUTRITIONAL ANALYSIS (per serving):

Calories: 86 Protein: 6g Carbohydrates: 10g Fat: 3g Saturated Fat: 1g Cholesterol: 9mg
Sodium: 185mg Fiber: 2g PCF Ratio: 25-43-32 Exchange Approx.: ½ Starch, 1 Vegetable, 1 Fat

INGREDIENTS | SERVES 6

1–3 slices bacon, cut into 1" pieces

1 tablespoon onion, chopped

2 cloves garlic, minced

1 tablespoon tomato paste

3 cups water

1 cup eggplant, peeled and cubed

¾ teaspoon salt

¼ teaspoon pepper

½ teaspoon oregano

8 ounces broccoli florets

1 cup whole-grain pasta shells, cooked al dente

1 ounce Romano cheese, grated

1. Place bacon, onion, and garlic in a 4-quart soup pot; brown.

2. Add tomato paste, water, eggplant, salt, pepper, and oregano. Bring to a boil; reduce heat and simmer for 20 minutes, or until eggplant is soft cooked.

3. Add broccoli florets; simmer for 5 minutes, until broccoli is tender but still slightly crisp. Add cooked pasta.

4. Serve soup immediately with a sprinkling of grated cheese.

Cold Roasted Red Pepper Soup

NUTRITIONAL ANALYSIS (per serving, without salt):

Calories: 73 Protein: 5g Carbohydrates: 9g Fat: 4g Saturated Fat: 1g Cholesterol: 3mg Sodium: 404mg
Fiber: 3g PCF Ratio: 21-39-40 Exchange Approx.: ½ Fat, ½ Starch

INGREDIENTS | SERVES 4

1 teaspoon olive oil

½ cup chopped onion

3 roasted red bell peppers, seeded and chopped (see Chapter 16)

3¼ cups low-fat, reduced-sodium chicken broth

½ cup nonfat plain yogurt

½ teaspoon sea salt (optional)

4 sprigs fresh basil (optional)

1. Heat saucepan over medium-high heat. Add olive oil; sauté onion until transparent. Add peppers and broth. Bring to a boil; reduce heat and simmer for 15 minutes. Remove from heat; purée in blender or food processor until smooth.

2. Allow to cool. Stir in yogurt and salt, if using; chill well in refrigerator. Garnish the soup with fresh basil sprigs, if desired.

Nutty Greek Snapper Soup

NUTRITIONAL ANALYSIS (per serving):

Calories: 309   Protein: 39g   Carbohydrates: 25g   Fat: 6g   Saturated Fat: 1g   Cholesterol: 46mg
Sodium: 240mg   Fiber: 2g   PCF Ratio: 50-33-17   Exchange Approx.: 4 Lean Meats, 1 Skim Milk, 1 Vegetable

INGREDIENTS | SERVES 4

1 pound (16 ounces) red snapper fillet

2 large cucumbers

4 green onions, chopped

4 cups nonfat plain yogurt

1 cup packed fresh parsley, basil, cilantro, arugula, and chives, mixed

3 tablespoons lime juice

Salt and pepper, to taste (optional)

¼ cup chopped walnuts

Herb sprigs for garnish (optional)

Tip

You can make this soup using leftover fish or substitute halibut, cod, or sea bass for the snapper.

1. Rinse red snapper fillet and pat dry with paper towels. Broil fillet until opaque through the thickest part, about 4 minutes on each side depending on the thickness of fillet. Let cool. (Alternatives would be to steam or poach the fillets.)

2. Peel and halve cucumbers and scoop out and discard seeds; cut into 1" pieces. Put half of cucumber with green onions in bowl of food processor; pulse to coarsely chop. Transfer to a large bowl.

3. Add remaining cucumber, yogurt, and herb leaves to food processor; process until smooth and frothy. (Alternatively, you can grate cucumbers, finely mince green onion and herbs, and stir together with yogurt in large bowl.) Stir in lime juice and season with salt and pepper to taste, if using. Cover and refrigerate for at least 1 hour, or up to 8 hours; the longer the soup cools, the more the flavors will mellow.

4. While soup cools, break cooled red snapper fillet into large chunks, discarding skin and any bones. Ladle chilled soup into shallow bowls and add red snapper. Sprinkle chopped walnuts over soup, garnish with herb sprigs, and serve.

White Bean and Escarole Soup

NUTRITIONAL ANALYSIS (per serving):

Calories: 163   Protein: 11g   Carbohydrates: 27g   Fat: 2g   Saturated Fat: 0g   Cholesterol: 7mg   Sodium: 349mg
Fiber: 9g   PCF Ratio: 26-64-10   Exchange Approx.: 1½ Starches, ½ Vegetable, 1½ Very-Lean Meats, 2 Fats

INGREDIENTS | SERVES 6

1 cup dry navy beans

3 cups water

1 cup onion, chopped

½ cup potato, peeled and chopped

1 clove garlic, minced

3 ounces Canadian bacon, cut in ½" cubes

2½ cups water

¼ teaspoon pepper

½ teaspoon salt

1 teaspoon vegetable oil

8 ounces escarole, coarsely chopped

1. Place dry beans and 3 cups of water in medium saucepan. Bring to a boil; remove from heat. Allow beans to soak several hours or overnight.

2. Drain beans; place in pressure cooker with onion, potatoes, garlic, Canadian bacon, 2½ cups water, salt, pepper, and vegetable oil. Close cover securely, place pressure regulator on vent pipe, and cook for 30 minutes with pressure regulator rocking slowly. (If using an electric pressure cooker, follow manufacturer instructions.) Let pressure drop on its own.

3. Add chopped escarole; simmer for 5–10 minutes, until escarole is wilted and cooked tender.

Slow-Cooker Method

This soup can also be prepared using a slow cooker. Soak beans as described in step 1; drain. Add beans, onion, potatoes, garlic, Canadian bacon, and 2½ cups water to slow cooker. Cook for 8–10 hours. At end of cooking, add escarole; simmer for 5–10 minutes, until escarole is wilted and tender. Add salt and pepper to taste.

Fresh Tomato Basil Soup

NUTRITIONAL ANALYSIS (per serving):

Calories: 87   Protein: 3g   Carbohydrates: 12g   Fat: 4g   Saturated Fat: 2g   Cholesterol: 10mg   Sodium: 449mg
Fiber: 3g   PCF Ratio: 13-50-37   Exchange Approx.: 2 Vegetables, 1 Fat

INGREDIENTS | SERVES 6

1 tablespoon butter

¼ cup onion, chopped

4 cups (2 pounds) crushed tomatoes

¼ cup fresh basil leaves, loosely chopped

1 cup low-sodium chicken broth

2 ounces reduced-fat (Neufchâtel) cream cheese

Fresh ground pepper, to taste

1. Melt butter in soup pot. Add onions; sauté until soft. Add crushed tomato, basil, and chicken broth.

2. Bring to a boil. Reduce heat; cook for another 15 minutes. Remove from heat; stir in cream cheese until melted.

3. Transfer to food processor or blender; purée until smooth. Depending on size of processor or blender, you may need to purée a partial portion at a time.

Winter Squash and Red Pepper Soup

NUTRITIONAL ANALYSIS (per serving):

Calories: 137   Protein: 3g   Carbohydrates: 24g   Fat: 3g   Saturated Fat: 1g   Cholesterol: 0mg
Sodium: 445mg   Fiber: 6g   PCF Ratio: 10-70-20   Exchange Approx.: 1 Starch, 1 Vegetable, ½ Fat

INGREDIENTS | SERVES 6

3½ cups winter squash, cooked

1 tablespoon olive oil

1 cup onions, chopped

1 tablespoon garlic, chopped

4 ounces roasted red pepper

3 cups low-sodium chicken broth

½ cup dry white wine

2 teaspoons sugar

1 teaspoon cinnamon

½ teaspoon ginger

1 tablespoon reduced-fat sour cream (optional)

1. Wash and cut squash in half; core out seeds. Place face down on oiled 9" × 13" glass baking dish; bake at 400°F for 50–60 minutes, or until squash is cooked tender. When cool enough to handle, scoop squash out of shells and set aside.

2. In large nonstick skillet heat, olive oil. Add onions and garlic; sauté until tender and continue to cook until the onions are soft and have turned brown (caramelized).

3. Add roasted pepper and chicken broth; simmer for another 16 minutes.

4. Add cooked winter squash, white wine, sugar, cinnamon, and ginger; simmer for another 5 minutes.

5. Transfer to food processor or blender; purée until smooth. Depending on size of processor or blender, you may need to purée a partial portion at a time. If desired, stir in reduced-fat sour cream and serve.

Rich and Creamy Sausage-Potato Soup

NUTRITIONAL ANALYSIS (per serving):

Calories: 326   Protein: 17g   Carbohydrates: 53g   Fat: 6g   Saturated Fat: 2g
Cholesterol: 19mg   Sodium: 259mg   Fiber: 3g   PCF Ratio: 20-64-16
Exchange Approx.:1 Fat, ½ Medium-Fat Meat, 1 Starch, 1½ Skim Milks, 1 Vegetable

INGREDIENTS | SERVES 2

1 teaspoon olive oil

½ teaspoon butter

½ cup chopped onion, steamed

1 clove dry roasted garlic (Chapter 10)

1 ounce crumbled cooked chorizo

¼ teaspoon celery seed

2 Yukon gold potatoes, peeled and diced into 1" pieces

½ cup fat-free chicken broth

1½ cups Mock Cream (Chapter 16)

1 teaspoon white wine vinegar

1 teaspoon vanilla extract

Optional seasonings to taste:

Fresh parsley

Sea salt and freshly ground black pepper

1. In saucepan, heat olive oil and butter over medium heat. Add onion, roasted garlic, chorizo, celery seed, and potatoes; sauté until heated.

2. Add chicken broth; bring to a boil. Cover saucepan, reduce heat, and maintain simmer for 10 minutes, or until potatoes are tender. Add Mock Cream and heat.

3. Remove pan from burner and stir in vinegar and vanilla.

Skim the Fat

You can remove fat from soups and stews by dropping ice cubes into the pot. The fat will cling to the cubes as you stir. Be sure to take out the cubes before they melt. Fat also clings to lettuce leaves; simply sweep them over the top of the soup. Discard ice cubes or leaves when done.

Chicken Corn Chowder

NUTRITIONAL ANALYSIS (per serving):

Calories: 193   Protein: 17g   Carbohydrates: 21g   Fat: 5g   Saturated Fat: 3g
Cholesterol: 39mg   Sodium: 155mg   Fiber: 2g   PCF Ratio: 22-36-42
Exchange Approx.: 1½ Very-Lean Meats, ½ Starch, 1 Vegetable, ½ Skim Milk, ½ High-Fat Meat

INGREDIENTS | SERVES 10

1 pound boneless, skinless chicken breast, cut into chunks

1 medium onion, chopped

1 red bell pepper, diced

1 large potato, diced

2 (16-ounce) cans low-fat, reduced-sodium chicken broth

1 (8¾-ounce) can unsalted cream-style corn

½ cup all-purpose flour

2 cups skim milk

4 ounces Cheddar cheese, diced

½ teaspoon sea salt

Freshly ground pepper, to taste

½ cup processed bacon bits

1. Spray large soup pot with nonstick cooking spray; heat on medium setting until hot. Add chicken, onion, and bell pepper; sauté over medium heat until chicken is browned and vegetables are tender. Stir in potatoes and broth; bring to a boil. Reduce heat and simmer, covered, for 20 minutes. Stir in corn.

2. Blend flour and milk in bowl; gradually stir into pot. Increase heat to medium; cook until mixture comes to a boil, then reduce heat and simmer until soup is thickened, stirring constantly. Add cheese; stir until melted and blended in. Add salt and pepper to taste and sprinkle with bacon bits before serving.

Tip

To trim down the fat in this recipe, use a reduced-fat cheese, such as Cabot's 50 Percent Light Cheddar.

Salmon Chowder

NUTRITIONAL ANALYSIS (per serving):

Calories: 364   Protein: 20g   Carbohydrates: 61g   Fat: 6g   Saturated Fat: 2g   Cholesterol: 28mg   Sodium: 199mg
Fiber: 7g   PCF Ratio: 22-65-14   Exchange Approx.: ½ Fat, 2 Starches, 2 Lean Meats, 2 Vegetables, ½ Skim Milk

INGREDIENTS | SERVES 4

1 (7½-ounce) can unsalted salmon

2 teaspoons butter

1 medium onion, chopped

2 stalks celery, chopped

1 sweet green pepper, seeded and chopped

1 clove garlic, minced

4 carrots, peeled and diced

4 small potatoes, peeled and diced

1 cup fat-free chicken broth

1 cup water

½ teaspoon cracked black pepper

½ teaspoon dill seed

1 cup diced zucchini

1 cup Mock Cream (Chapter 16)

1 (8¾-ounce) can unsalted cream-style corn

Freshly ground black pepper, to taste

½ cup chopped fresh parsley (optional)

1. Drain and flake salmon; discard liquid.

2. In large nonstick saucepan, melt butter over medium heat; sauté onion, celery, green pepper, garlic, and carrots, stirring often, until tender, about 5 minutes.

3. Add potatoes, broth, water, pepper, and dill seed; bring to boil. Reduce heat, cover, and simmer for 20 minutes, or until potatoes are tender.

4. Add zucchini; simmer, covered, for another 5 minutes.

5. Add salmon, Mock Cream, corn, and pepper; cook over low heat just until heated through. Just before serving, add parsley, if desired.

CHAPTER 9

Meat Dishes

Beef Broth: Easy Slow-Cooker Method

NUTRITIONAL ANALYSIS (per serving):

Calories: 58   Protein: 9g   Carbohydrates: 0g   Fat: 2g   Saturated Fat: 1g   Cholesterol: 27mg   Sodium: 14mg
Fiber: 0g   PCF Ratio: 65-0-35   Exchange Approx.: 1 Lean Meat

INGREDIENTS | YIELDS ABOUT 3 CUPS BROTH; SERVING SIZE: ½ CUP

1 pound lean round steak
1 onion, chopped
2 carrots, peeled and chopped
2 celery stalks and leaves, chopped
1 bay leaf
4 sprigs parsley
6 black peppercorns
¼ cup dry white wine
4½ cups water

Trade Secrets

Some chefs swear that a hearty beef broth requires oven-roasted bones. Place bones on a roasting tray and bake in 425°F oven for 30–60 minutes. Blot fat from bones before adding to rest of broth ingredients. You may need to reduce amount of water in your slow cooker, which will produce a more concentrated broth.

1. Cut beef into several pieces; add to slow cooker with all other ingredients. Use high setting until mixture reaches a boil, then reduce heat to low. Allow to simmer, covered, overnight, or up to 16 hours.

2. Remove beef and drain on paper towels to absorb any fat. Strain broth, discarding meat and vegetables. (You don't want to eat vegetables cooked directly with the beef because they will have absorbed too much of the residue fat.) Put broth in a covered container and refrigerate for several hours or overnight; this allows time for fat to congeal on top of broth. Remove hardened fat and discard. (When you remove fat from broth, the Exchange Approximation for it will be a Free Exchange.) Broth will keep in refrigerator for a few days. Freeze any you won't use within that time.

Stovetop Grilled Beef Loin

NUTRITIONAL ANALYSIS (per serving):

Calories: 105   Protein: 15g   Carbohydrates: 1g   Fat: 4g   Saturated Fat: 1g   Cholesterol: 2mg
Sodium: 27mg   Fiber: 0g   PCF Ratio: 58-5-37   Exchange Approx.: 2½ Lean Meats

INGREDIENTS | YIELDS 1 (5-OUNCE) LOIN; SERVING SIZE: 2½ OUNCES

1 lean beef tenderloin fillet, no more than 1" thick

½ teaspoon paprika

1½ teaspoons garlic powder

⅛ teaspoon cracked black pepper

¼ teaspoon onion powder

Pinch to ⅛ teaspoon cayenne pepper (according to taste)

⅛ teaspoon dried oregano

⅛ teaspoon dried thyme

½ teaspoon brown sugar

½ teaspoon olive oil

Weights and Measures: Before and After

Exchanges are based on cooking weight of meats; however, in the case of lean pork loin trimmed of all fat, very little weight is lost during the cooking process. Therefore, amounts given for raw pork loin in recipes equal cooked weights. If you find your cooking method causes more variation in weight, adjust accordingly.

1. Remove loin from refrigerator 30 minutes before preparing it to allow it to come to room temperature. Pat meat dry with paper towels.

2. Mix together all dry ingredients. Rub ¼ teaspoon of olive oil on each side of the fillet. (The olive oil is used in this recipe to help the "rub" adhere to the meat and to aid in the caramelization process.) Divide seasoning mixture; rub into each oiled side.

3. Heat a grill pan on high for 1–2 minutes, until the pan is sizzling hot. Place beef fillet in pan, reduce heat to medium-high, and cook 3 minutes. Use tongs to turn fillet. (Be careful not to pierce meat.) Cook for another 2 minutes for medium or 3 minutes for well-done.

4. Remove from heat and let the meat rest in pan for at least 5 minutes, allowing juices to redistribute throughout meat and complete cooking process, which makes for a juicier fillet.

The Ultimate Grilled Cheeseburger Sandwich

NUTRITIONAL ANALYSIS (per serving):

Calories: 262 Protein: 17g Carbohydrates: 15g Fat: 15g Saturated Fat: 5g Cholesterol: 60mg
Sodium: 252mg Fiber: 1.22g PCF Ratio: 26-24-50 Exchange Approx.: 2 Lean Meats, 1 Fat, 1 Starch

INGREDIENTS | SERVES 4

1 tablespoon olive oil

1 teaspoon butter

2 thick slices of 7-Grain Bread (Chapter 18)

1 ounce Cheddar cheese

½ pound (8 ounces) ground round

1 teaspoon Worcestershire sauce, or to taste

Fresh minced garlic, to taste

Balsamic vinegar, to taste

Toppings of your choice such as stoneground mustard, mayonnaise, etc.

The Olive Oil Factor

Once you've used an olive oil and butter mixture to butter the bread for a toasted or grilled sandwich, you'll never want to use just plain butter again! Olive oil helps make the bread crunchier and imparts a subtle taste difference to the sandwiches.

1. Preheat indoor grill. Combine olive oil and butter; use ½ to butter 1 side of each slice of bread. Place Cheddar cheese on unbuttered side of 1 slice of bread; top with other slice, buttered-side up.

2. Combine ground round with Worcestershire sauce, garlic, and balsamic vinegar, if using. Shape ground round into large, rectangular patty, a little larger than slice of bread. Grill patty and then cheese sandwich. (If you are using a large indoor grill, position hamburger at lower end, near area where fat drains; grill cheese sandwich at higher end.)

3. Once cheese sandwich is done, separate slices of bread, being careful not to burn yourself on cheese. Top 1 slice with hamburger and add your choice of condiments and fixin's.

Southwest Black Bean Burgers

NUTRITIONAL ANALYSIS (per serving):

Calories: 230   Protein: 20g   Carbohydrates: 10g   Fat: 12g   Saturated Fat: 4g   Cholesterol: 55mg
Sodium: 15.02mg   Fiber: 4g   PCF Ratio: 36-18-46   Exchange Approx.: 2½ Lean Meats, ½ Starch, 1 Fat

INGREDIENTS | SERVES 5

1 cup black beans, cooked

¼ cup onion, chopped

1 teaspoon chili powder

1 teaspoon ground cumin

1 tablespoon fresh parsley, minced

1 tablespoon fresh cilantro, minced

½ teaspoon salt (optional)

¾ pound lean ground beef

Swapping Fresh Herbs for Dried

If you do not have fresh herbs such as parsley or cilantro available, 1 teaspoon dried can be used in place of 1 tablespoon fresh.

1. Place beans, onion, chili powder, cumin, parsley, cilantro, and salt in food processor. Combine ingredients using pulse setting until beans are partially puréed and all ingredients are mixed. (If using canned beans, drain and rinse first.)

2. In a separate bowl, combine ground beef and bean mixture. Shape into 5 patties.

3. Meat mixture is quite soft after mixing and should be chilled or partially frozen prior to cooking. Grill or broil on oiled surface.

Italian Sausage

NUTRITIONAL ANALYSIS (per serving, without salt):

Calories: 135   Protein: 15g   Carbohydrates: 0g   Fat: 8g   Saturated Fat: 3g   Cholesterol: 45mg
Sodium: 27mg   Fiber: 0g   PCF Ratio: 47-0-53   Exchange Approx.: 1 Medium-Fat Meat

INGREDIENTS | YIELDS ABOUT 2 POUNDS (32 OUNCES); SERVING SIZE: 2 OUNCES

2 pounds (32 ounces) pork shoulder

1 teaspoon ground black pepper

1 teaspoon dried parsley

1 teaspoon Italian-style seasoning

1 teaspoon garlic powder

¾ teaspoon crushed anise seeds

⅛ teaspoon crushed red pepper flakes

½ teaspoon paprika

½ teaspoon instant minced onion flakes

1 teaspoon kosher or sea salt (optional)

Simple (and Smart!) Substitutions

Game meats—buffalo, venison, elk, moose—are low in fat, as are ground chicken or turkey. Substitute one of these for pork in any of the sausage recipes in this chapter.

1. Remove all fat from meat; cut the meat into cubes. Put in food processor; grind to desired consistency.

2. Add remaining ingredients; mix until well blended. You can put sausage mixture in casings, but it works equally well broiled or grilled as patties.

Italian Sweet Fennel Sausage

NUTRITIONAL ANALYSIS (per serving, without salt):

Calories: 139   Protein: 15g   Carbohydrates: 1g   Fat: 8g   Saturated Fat: 3g   Cholesterol: 45mg
Sodium: 27mg   Fiber: 0g   PCF Ratio: 46-3-51   Exchange Approx.: 1 Medium-Fat Meat

INGREDIENTS | YIELDS ABOUT 2 POUNDS (32 OUNCES); SERVING SIZE: 2 OUNCES

2 pounds (32 ounces) pork butt
½ teaspoon black pepper
2½ teaspoons crushed garlic
1 tablespoon sugar
1 teaspoon kosher or sea salt (optional)

1. Toast fennel seeds and cayenne pepper in nonstick skillet over medium heat, stirring constantly, until seeds just begin to darken, about 2 minutes. Set aside.

2. Remove all fat from meat; cut the meat into cubes. Put in food processor; grind to desired consistency. Add remaining ingredients; mix until well blended. You can put sausage mixture in casings, but it works equally well broiled or grilled as patties.

Better the Second Day

Ideally, sausage is made the night before and refrigerated to allow the flavors to merge. Leftover sausage can be frozen for up to 3 months.

Mock Chorizo

NUTRITIONAL ANALYSIS (per serving, without salt):

Calories: 137   Protein: 15g   Carbohydrates: 1g   Fat: 8g   Saturated Fat: 3g   Cholesterol: 45mg
Sodium: 27mg   Fiber: 0g   PCF Ratio: 47-1-52   Exchange Approx.: 1 Medium-Fat Meat

INGREDIENTS | YIELDS ABOUT 2 POUNDS (32 OUNCES); SERVING SIZE: 2 OUNCES

2 pounds (32 ounces) lean pork

4 tablespoons chili powder

¼ teaspoon ground cloves

2 tablespoons paprika

2½ teaspoons crushed fresh garlic

1 teaspoon crushed dried oregano

3½ tablespoons cider vinegar

1 teaspoon kosher or sea salt (optional)

1. Remove all fat from meat; cut the meat into cubes. Put in food processor; grind to desired consistency. Add remaining ingredients; mix until well blended.

2. Tradition calls for aging this sausage in an airtight container in the refrigerator for 4 days before cooking. Leftover sausage can be stored in the freezer up to 3 months.

Break from Tradition

Traditionally, chorizo is very high in fat. This chorizo recipe is a lower-fat alternative. It makes an excellent replacement for adding flavor to recipes that call for bacon. In fact, 1 or 2 ounces of chorizo can replace an entire pound of bacon in cabbage, bean, or potato soup.

Kousa (Squash Stuffed with Lamb and Rice)

NUTRITIONAL ANALYSIS:

Calories: 430   Protein: 27g   Carbohydrates: 36g   Fat: 20g   Saturated Fat: 7g   Cholesterol: 82mg
Sodium: 692mg   Fiber: 5g   PCF Ratio: 25-33-42   Exchange Approx.: 3 Lean Meats, 1 Starch, 3 Vegetables, 3 Fats

INGREDIENTS | SERVES 4

3 cups tomatoes, chopped

1 cup onion, chopped

2 cups water

½ teaspoon salt

⅛ teaspoon fresh ground pepper

2 tablespoons fresh mint, minced

4 small zucchini squash (7"–8" long)

¾ pound very lean ground lamb

½ cup rice

2 tablespoons pine nuts

½ teaspoon salt

⅛ teaspoon allspice

⅛ teaspoon fresh ground pepper

Summer Harvest

Kousa (stuffed squash) is a traditional Lebanese dish that uses a pale green summer squash very similar to zucchini. This squash is not always easy to find, but zucchini is very abundant and works quite well. If you have a large garden crop of zucchini: pick them small, hollow out the squash, blanch in boiling water for 2 minutes, then freeze. You'll have squash ready to stuff all year long.

1. Prepare tomato sauce first: Combine tomatoes, onion, water, salt, pepper, and fresh mint in a large pot. Bring to a boil; reduce heat and simmer 30 minutes.

2. Scrub squash and dry with paper towels. Remove stem ends of each squash and carefully core center, leaving about ¼" of shell.

3. Make stuffing: thoroughly mix ground lamb, rice, pine nuts, salt, allspice, and pepper.

4. Spoon stuffing into each squash, tapping bottom end of squash to get stuffing down. Fill each squash to top; stuffing should be loosely packed to allow rice to expand while cooking.

5. Place squash in tomato sauce, laying them on their sides. Bring sauce to a slow boil; cover and cook over low heat for 45–60 minutes, or until squash is tender and rice has cooked. Serve squash with tomato sauce spooned over top.

Baked Stuffed Kibbeh (Ground Lamb and Bulgur Wheat)

NUTRITIONAL ANALYSIS:

Calories: 226   Protein: 18g   Carbohydrates: 13g   Fat: 12g   Saturated Fat: 4g   Cholesterol: 62mg
Sodium: 343mg   Fiber: 3g   PCF Ratio: 32-22-46   Exchange Approx.: 1 Starch, 2 Lean Meats, 2 Fats

INGREDIENTS | SERVES 8

Cooking spray
¾ cup bulgur wheat, fine grind
2 cups boiling water
1 pound lean ground lamb
1 cup onion, grated
1 teaspoon salt
¼ teaspoon pepper
Small bowl ice water
1½ tablespoons butter, melted
¼ cup pine nuts
¼ teaspoon cinnamon
¼ teaspoon allspice
1½ tablespoons butter, melted

Making Lean Ground Lamb

Unless you have a butcher, very lean ground lamb is difficult to find. Make it yourself using chunks of meat trimmed from a leg of lamb. Be sure to remove all visible fat from the lamb and grind twice using a medium or fine grinder blade. Removing all visible fat prevents lamb from having a strong "mutton" taste.

1. Spray 9" × 9" baking dish with cooking spray.

2. Put bulgur wheat in small bowl. Cover with boiling water and allow wheat to absorb liquid, approximately 15–20 minutes.

3. Line colander with small piece of cheesecloth. Drop bulgur wheat into cloth; drain and squeeze as much liquid out of wheat as possible.

4. On large cutting board, combine lamb, ½ grated onions, wheat, salt, and pepper; mix with hands, kneading together all ingredients.

5. Divide meat mixture in ½. Place ½ in bottom of baking dish by dipping hands into ice water to spread meat mixture smoothly over bottom of dish. Cover bottom of dish completely.

6. In a small pan, melt 1½ tablespoons of butter; sauté remaining onions, pine nuts, cinnamon, and allspice until onions are soft.

7. Spread onion and pine nut mixture evenly over first layer of meat in baking dish. Take remaining ½ of meat mixture and spread smoothly on top, using procedure in step 5.

8. Score top in diamond shapes with a knife dipped in cold water. Melt remaining 1½ tablespoons of butter; drizzle over top of meat. Bake at 350°F for approximately 40–45 minutes, or until gold brown.

Slow-Cooker Beef Braciole

NUTRITIONAL ANALYSIS (per serving):

Calories: 367   Protein: 29g   Carbohydrates: 25.93g   Fat: 16g   Saturated Fat: 5g   Cholesterol: 69mg   Sodium: 162mg
Fiber: 5g   PCF Ratio: 32-29-39   Exchange Approx.: 3½ Very-Lean Meats, 2½ Fats, 3 Vegetables, 1 Starch

INGREDIENTS | SERVES 4

4 cups tomato sauce

1 tablespoon olive oil

¼ cup onion, finely chopped

1 teaspoon garlic, finely chopped

¼ cup carrots, finely chopped

¼ cup celery, finely chopped

2 slices whole-wheat bread, cubed

1 egg, lightly beaten

1 pound thinly sliced round beef, cut into 4 pieces

1. Prepare tomato sauce in slow cooker (see Chapter 13 or use your own sauce recipe) in advance and maintain at medium heat.

2. Heat olive oil in large nonstick skillet; sauté onions, garlic, carrots and celery until softened. Remove from heat.

3. Add cubed bread and egg to sautéed vegetables; mix well.

4. Pound each piece of beef on both sides to flatten and tenderize. Each slice of meat should be about ¼" thick. Place approximately ½ cup of bread and vegetable stuffing down center of each meat slice and press in place. Starting at one end, roll meat up like a jelly roll; secure with 6" wooden skewer.

5. Place meat rolls in tomato sauce. Set slow cooker on low to medium setting; cook for at least 4 hours. (On low setting, the meat rolls can be left in slow cooker for 6–8 hours.) Remove wooden skewers before serving.

Soy and Ginger Flank Steak

NUTRITIONAL ANALYSIS (per serving):

Calories: 304   Protein: 29g   Carbohydrates: 1g   Fat: 19g   Saturated Fat: 7g   Cholesterol: 95mg
Sodium: 213mg   Fiber: 0g   PCF Ratio: 40-2-58   Exchange Approx.: 4 Lean Meats, 1½ Fats

INGREDIENTS | SERVES 4

1 pound lean London broil
1 tablespoon fresh ginger, minced
2 teaspoons fresh garlic, minced
1 tablespoon reduced-sodium soy sauce
3 tablespoons dry red wine
¼ teaspoon pepper
½ tablespoon olive oil

Slicing Meats Against the Grain

Certain cuts of meat such as flank steak, brisket, and London broil have a distinct grain (or line) of fibers running through them. If you slice with the grain, meat will seem tough and difficult to chew. These cuts of meat should always be thinly sliced across (or against) the grain so fibers are cut through so meats remain tender and easy to chew.

1. Marinate meat at least 3–4 hours in advance. Place meat, ginger, garlic, soy sauce, red wine, pepper, and olive oil in shallow baking dish. Coat meat with marinade on both sides.

2. Cover and refrigerate meat in marinade, turning meat once or twice during marinating so all marinade soaks into both sides of meat.

3. Lightly oil barbecue grill and preheat. Place flank steak on grill. Grill steak, turning once, until done to your preference. Medium-rare will take approximately 12–15 minutes. Slice meat diagonally and against grain into thin slices.

Pork Lo Mein

NUTRITIONAL ANALYSIS (per serving):

Calories: 266   Protein: 23g   Carbohydrates: 25g   Fat: 8g   Saturated Fat: 2g   Cholesterol: 50mg
Sodium: 386mg   Fiber: 5g   PCF Ratio: 35-38-27   Exchange Approx.: 2½ Lean Meats, 1 Starch, 1 Vegetable

INGREDIENTS | SERVES 4

1½ tablespoons reduced-sodium soy sauce

1 teaspoon fresh ginger, grated

1 tablespoon rice vinegar

¼ teaspoon turmeric

¾ pound lean pork loin, cut into 1" cubes

½ cup green onion, sliced

2 teaspoons garlic, minced

2 cups cabbage, shredded

1 cup snap peas, cut into 1" pieces

½ tablespoon canola oil

¼ teaspoon crushed red pepper

2 cups whole-grain spaghetti, cooked

1 teaspoon sesame oil

1 teaspoon sesame seeds

1. Combine soy sauce, ginger, rice vinegar, and turmeric in bowl. Mix in cubed pork; set aside.

2. Cut up onion, garlic, cabbage, and snap peas before starting stir-fry.

3. In large skillet or wok, heat oil and sauté onion and garlic. Add meat; cook quickly until meat and onions are slightly browned.

4. Add in cabbage and snap peas; continue to stir-fry for another 3–4 minutes. Sprinkle in crushed red pepper.

5. When vegetables are crisp-tender, add cooked pasta, sesame oil, and sesame seeds. Toss lightly and serve.

Pork Roast with Caramelized Onions and Apples

NUTRITIONAL ANALYSIS (per serving):

Calories: 373   Protein: 31g   Carbohydrates: 8g   Fat: 23g   Saturated Fat: 9g   Cholesterol: 96mg
Sodium: 156mg   Fiber: 1g   PCF Ratio: 34-9-57   Exchange Approx.: 1 Vegetable, 4 Lean Meats, 2 Fats

INGREDIENTS | SERVES 6

2 pounds lean pork loin roast

Fresh ground pepper, to taste

½ tablespoon olive oil

½ tablespoon butter

2 cups onion, chopped

1 tablespoon Marsala wine

⅓ cup low-sodium chicken broth

1 apple, peeled and chopped

1. Preheat oven to 375°F. Season pork loin with pepper. Heat olive oil in a large skillet; sear to brown all sides.

2. Transfer roast to 9" × 13" glass baking dish; place in oven for approximately 1 hour and 15 minutes.

3. While pork is roasting, prepare onions: In large nonstick skillet, melt butter and add onions. Sauté onions until soft; add wine, chicken broth, and apple. Continue cooking on low heat until onions are soft, brown in color, and have caramelized.

4. When roast has reached an internal temperature of 130°F, spoon onions over top; place a loose foil tent over roast.

5. Remove roast from oven when an internal temperature of 145°F has been reached. (Temperature of roast will continue to rise as meat rests.) Keep roast loosely covered with foil and allow to stand for 10–15 minutes before slicing.

Fruited Pork Loin Roast Casserole

NUTRITIONAL ANALYSIS (per serving):

Calories: 170   Protein: 7g   Carbohydrates: 27g   Fat: 4g   Saturated Fat: 1g   Cholesterol: 19mg
Sodium: 32mg   Fiber: 3g   PCF Ratio: 17-63-20   Exchange Approx.: 1 Lean Meat, 1 Fruit, 1 Starch

INGREDIENTS | SERVES 4

4 small Yukon Gold potatoes, peeled and sliced

2 (2-ounce) pieces trimmed boneless pork loin, pounded flat

1 apple, peeled, cored, and sliced

4 apricot halves

1 tablespoon chopped red onion or shallot

⅛ cup apple cider or apple juice

Optional seasonings, to taste:

Olive oil

Parmesan cheese

Salt and freshly ground pepper

1. Preheat oven to 350°F (325°F if using a glass casserole dish); treat casserole dish with nonstick spray.

2. Layer ½ of potato slices across bottom of dish; top with 1 piece of flattened pork loin. Arrange apple slices over top of loin; place apricot halves on top of apple. Sprinkle red onion over apricot and apples. Add second flattened pork loin; layer remaining potatoes atop loin. Drizzle apple cider overtop of casserole.

3. Cover and bake for 45 minutes to 1 hour, or until potatoes are tender. Keep casserole covered and let sit for 10 minutes after removing from oven.

Tip

To enhance the flavor of this dish, top with the optional ingredients when it's served. Just be sure to make the appropriate Exchange Approximations adjustments if you do.

White Wine and Lemon Pork Roast

NUTRITIONAL ANALYSIS (per serving):

Calories: 172   Protein: 18g   Carbohydrates: 2g   Fat: 7g   Saturated Fat: 2g   Cholesterol: 50mg
Sodium: 47mg   Fiber: 0g   PCF Ratio: 53-5-42   Exchange Approx.: 3 Lean Meats

INGREDIENTS | SERVES 4

1 clove garlic, crushed

½ cup dry white wine

1 tablespoon lemon juice

1 teaspoon olive oil

1 tablespoon minced red onion or shallot

¼ teaspoon dried thyme

⅛ teaspoon ground black pepper

12 ounces pork loin roast

1. Make marinade by combining garlic, white wine, lemon juice, olive oil, red onion, thyme, and black pepper in heavy, freezer-style plastic bag. Add roast; marinate in refrigerator 1 hour or overnight, according to taste. (Note: Pork loin is already tender, so you're marinating the meat to impart the flavors only.)

2. Preheat oven to 350°F. Remove meat from marinade; put on nonstick spray–treated rack in roasting pan. Roast for 20–30 minutes, or until meat thermometer reads 150°F to 170°F, depending on how well done you prefer it.

Marmalade Marinade

Combine 1 teaspoon Dijon or stone-ground mustard, 1 tablespoon Smucker's Low-Sugar Orange Marmalade, 1 clove crushed garlic, and ¼ teaspoon dried thyme leaves. Marinate and prepare a ½-pound (8-ounce) pork loin as you would the White Wine and Lemon Pork Loin Roast. The Nutritional Analysis for a 2-ounce serving is: Calories: 89.52; Protein: 12.26g; Carbohydrate: 1.90g; Fat: 3.26g; Saturated Fat: 1.11g; Cholesterol: 33.45mg; Sodium: 43.66mg; Fiber: 0.09g; PCF Ratio: 57-9-34; Exchange Approximations: 2 Lean Meats.

Balsamic Venison Pot Roast

NUTRITIONAL ANALYSIS (per serving):

Calories: 188   Protein: 28g   Carbohydrates: 6g   Fat: 6g   Saturated Fat: 2g   Cholesterol: 96mg
Sodium: 75mg   Fiber: 1g   PCF Ratio: 60-13-28   Exchange Approx.: 4 Very Lean Meats, ½ Fat

INGREDIENTS | SERVES 8

2½ tablespoons all-purpose flour

2 teaspoons paprika

2-pound venison roast

1½ tablespoons olive oil

14 ounces low-sodium beef broth

½ cup onion, chopped

2 tablespoons dried onion flakes

⅓ cup balsamic vinegar

⅛ teaspoon Worcestershire sauce

1 teaspoon sugar

Recipe Adaptation

This recipe also works well cooked in a slow cooker for 6–8 hours, until tender. Slow cookers with a ceramic interior maintain low temperatures better than those with a metal cooking surface.

1. Mix flour and paprika together; dredge venison in flour mixture and completely coat with flour.

2. Heat oil in Dutch oven or deep skillet; brown roast on all sides.

3. Add beef broth, onion, onion flakes, balsamic vinegar, Worcestershire sauce, and sugar. Bring to a quick boil; reduce heat to low.

4. Cover and cook over low heat for 2–3 hours, or until venison is tender and cuts easily. Serve with whole-grain noodles.

Venison Pepper Steak

NUTRITIONAL ANALYSIS (per serving):

Calories: 237   Protein: 26g   Carbohydrates: 12g   Fat: 9g   Saturated Fat: 3g   Cholesterol: 39mg
Sodium: 344mg   Fiber: 2g   PCF Ratio: 44-20-36   Exchange Approx.: 3½ Very-Lean Meats, 2 Vegetables, 1½ Fats

INGREDIENTS | SERVES 4

1 pound venison loin

2 tablespoons reduced-sodium soy sauce

1 clove garlic

1½ teaspoons ginger, grated

1 tablespoon canola oil

1 cup onion, thinly sliced

1 cup green or red peppers, cut into ½" strips

½ cup celery, thinly sliced

1 tablespoon cornstarch

1 cup water

1½ cups tomatoes, chopped

1. Cut meat across grain into ¼" strips.

2. Combine soy sauce, garlic, and ginger in bowl. Add sliced meat; mix well and set aside.

3. Heat canola oil in large wok or skillet. Add meat and cook for 2-3 minutes over high heat. Cover, reduce heat, and simmer for 15 minutes.

4. Add onions, peppers, and celery to meat; cover and cook on low heat for another 15 minutes, or until sliced meat is tender.

5. Mix cornstarch with water; add to meat. Cook for 5 minutes, or until sauce thickens slightly. Add tomatoes and heat through.

Whole Grain Additions

Instead of serving white rice, substitute brown rice or quinoa mixed with sautéed vegetables with this dish.

Slow-Cooker Venison and Vegetable Pot Roast

NUTRITIONAL ANALYSIS (per serving):

Calories: 309   Protein: 27g   Carbohydrates: 28g   Fat: 10g   Saturated Fat: 3g   Cholesterol: 39mg   Sodium: 237mg
Fiber: 4g   PCF Ratio: 35-36-28   Exchange Approx.: 3½ Very-Lean Meats, 1 Starch, 3 Vegetables, 1½ Fats

INGREDIENTS | SERVES 4

1-pound venison roast
1 tablespoon all-purpose flour
1 tablespoon olive oil
1 tablespoon instant brown gravy mix
1 teaspoon Worcestershire sauce
1 cup onions, chopped
½ pound potatoes, cut into 1" pieces
1 cup carrots, cut into 1" pieces
1 cup celery, chopped
½ cup crushed tomato
½ teaspoon dried thyme leaves

1. Dredge roast in flour. Heat olive oil in large skillet; sear roast until browned on all sides. Put roast in slow cooker.

2. Sprinkle instant gravy mix and Worcestershire sauce over top of roast. Place onions, potatoes, carrots, and celery around roast; spoon crushed tomatoes evenly around vegetables. Sprinkle thyme over meat and vegetables.

3. Cook in slow cooker on low setting for 6–8 hours.

Variation

You can also use ⅓ cup water and 2 tablespoons red wine for the liquid instead of crushed tomatoes.

CHAPTER 10

Poultry Dishes

Chicken Broth: Easy Slow-Cooker Method

NUTRITIONAL ANALYSIS (per serving):

Calories: 67   Protein: 9g   Carbohydrates: 0g   Fat: 3g   Saturated Fat: 1g   Cholesterol: 24mg   Sodium: 22mg   Fiber: 0g   PCF Ratio: 53-0-47   Exchange Approx.: ½ Very-Lean Meat, ½ Lean Meat

INGREDIENTS | YIELD ABOUT 4 CUPS; SERVING SIZE: ½ CUP

1 small onion, chopped

2 carrots, peeled and chopped

2 celery stalks and leaves, chopped

1 bay leaf

4 sprigs parsley

6 black peppercorns

¼ cup dry white wine

2 pounds chicken pieces, skin removed

4½ cups water

Reduced Broth

Reducing broth is the act of boiling it to decrease the amount of water so you're left with a richer broth. Boiling nonfat, canned chicken broth won't reduce it as a home-made broth would. The broth from this recipe will be richer than what most recipes call for, so unless you need reduced broth, thin it with water as needed. Assuming you remove the fat from the broth, it will be a Free Exchange.

1. Add all ingredients except water to slow cooker. The chicken pieces and vegetables should be loosely layered and fill no more than ¾ of slow cooker. Add enough water to just cover ingredients; cover slow cooker. Use high setting until mixture almost reaches a boil, then reduce heat to low. Allow to simmer overnight or up to 16 hours, checking occasionally and adding more water, if necessary.

2. Remove chicken pieces and drain on paper towels to absorb any fat. Allow to cool; remove meat from bones. Strain vegetables from broth and discard. (You don't want to eat vegetables cooked directly with chicken because they will have absorbed too much of the residue fat.) Put broth in a covered container; refrigerate for several hours or overnight, allowing fat to congeal on top. Remove hardened fat and discard.

3. To separate broth into small amounts for use when you steam vegetables or potatoes, fill up an ice cube tray with stock. Let freeze, then remove cubes from tray and store in labeled freezer bag. Common ice cube trays allow for ⅛ cup or 2 tablespoons of liquid per section.

Oven-Fried Chicken Thighs

NUTRITIONAL ANALYSIS (per serving, no oil):

Calories: 74   Protein: 9g   Carbohydrates: 5g   Fat: 2g   Saturated Fat: 1g   Cholesterol: 34mg
Sodium: 331mg   Fiber: 0g   PCF Ratio: 53-26-21   Exchange Approx.: 2 Very-Lean Meats

INGREDIENTS | SERVES 4

4 chicken thighs, skin removed

1 tablespoon unbleached, white all-purpose flour

1 large egg white

½ teaspoon sea salt

½ teaspoon olive oil (optional; see Comparison Analysis for using olive oil)

1 tablespoon rice flour

1 tablespoon cornmeal

If You Use Oil . . .
Comparison Analysis (with olive oil): Calories: 78.53; Protein: 9.46g; Carbohydrate: 4.65g; Fat: 2.27g; Saturated Fat: 0.50g; Cholesterol: 34.03mg; Sodium: 331.03mg; Fiber: 0.06g; PCF Ratio: 49-24-27; Exchange Approx.: 2 Lean Meats.

1. Preheat oven to 350°F. Rinse and dry chicken thighs. Put white flour on plate. In small, shallow bowl, whip egg white with the sea salt. Add olive oil, if using; mix well. Put rice flour and cornmeal on another plate; mix together. Place rack on baking sheet; spray both with nonstick cooking spray.

2. Roll each chicken thigh in white flour, dip it into egg mixture, and roll in rice flour mixture. Place thighs on rack so they aren't touching. Bake 35–45 minutes, until meat juices run clear.

Another Healthy "Fried" Chicken

NUTRITIONAL ANALYSIS (per serving):

Calories: 118   Protein: 19g   Carbohydrates: 5g   Fat: 2g   Saturated Fat: 1g   Cholesterol: 44mg
Sodium: 91mg   Fiber: 0g   PCF Ratio: 66-18-16   Exchange Approx.: 2 Very-Lean Meats, ½ Starch

INGREDIENTS | SERVES 4

10 ounces raw boneless, skinless chicken breasts (fat trimmed off)

½ cup nonfat plain yogurt

½ cup bread crumbs

1 teaspoon garlic powder

1 teaspoon paprika

¼ teaspoon dried thyme

Chicken Fat Facts

When faced with the decision of whether to have chicken with or without the skin, consider that ½ pound of skinless chicken breast has 9g of fat; ½ pound with the skin on has 38g!

1. Preheat oven to 350°F. Prepare baking pan with nonstick cooking spray. Cut chicken breast into 4 equal pieces; marinate in yogurt for several minutes.

2. Mix together bread crumbs, garlic, paprika, and thyme; dredge chicken in crumb mixture. Arrange on prepared pan; bake 20 minutes. To give chicken a deep golden color, place pan under broiler last 5 minutes of cooking. Watch closely to ensure chicken "crust" doesn't burn.

Buttermilk Ranch Chicken Salad

NUTRITIONAL ANALYSIS (per serving):

Calories: 147 Protein: 18g Carbohydrates: 11g Fat: 4g Saturated Fat: 1g Cholesterol: 33mg Sodium: 184mg
Fiber: 2g PCF Ratio: 49-29-22 Exchange Approx.: 2 Very-Lean Meats, ½ Vegetable, 1 Free Vegetable, ½ Skim Milk

INGREDIENTS | SERVES 4

1 tablespoon real mayonnaise

3 tablespoons nonfat plain yogurt

½ cup nonfat cottage cheese

½ teaspoon cider vinegar

1 teaspoon brown sugar

1 teaspoon Dijon mustard

½ cup buttermilk

2 tablespoons dried parsley

1 clove garlic, minced

2 tablespoons grated Parmesan cheese

¼ teaspoon sea salt (optional)

¼ teaspoon freshly ground pepper (optional)

1 cup chopped cooked chicken breast

½ cup sliced cucumber

½ cup chopped celery

½ cup sliced carrots

4 cups salad greens

½ cup red onion slices

Fresh parsley for garnish (optional)

1. In blender or food processor, combine mayonnaise, yogurt, cottage cheese, vinegar, brown sugar, mustard, buttermilk, parsley, garlic, cheese, salt, and pepper; process until smooth. Pour over the chicken, cucumber, celery, and carrots. Chill at least 2 hours.

2. To serve, arrange 1 cup of salad greens on each of 4 serving plates. Top each salad with an equal amount of chicken salad. Garnish with red onion slices and fresh parsley, if desired.

Get More Mileage from Your Meals

Leftover Chicken Salad makes great sandwiches. Put it between two slices of bread with lots of lettuce for a quick lunch. The lettuce helps keep the bread from getting soggy if the sandwich is to go.

Pineapple-Orange Grilled Chicken Breasts

NUTRITIONAL ANALYSIS (per serving):

Calories: 165   Protein: 27g   Carbohydrates: 10g   Fat: 2g   Saturated Fat: 0g   Cholesterol: 58.40mg
Sodium: 75mg   Fiber: 0g   PCF Ratio: 67-25-9   Exchange Approx.: 3½ Lean Meats, ½ Fruit

INGREDIENTS | SERVES 4

6 ounces pineapple juice

4 ounces orange juice

¼ cup cider vinegar

1 tablespoon fresh tarragon, chopped

½ tablespoon fresh rosemary

1 pound boneless chicken breast, skinned and cut into 4 pieces

1. Mix marinade in large shallow dish 3-4 hours before grilling: pineapple juice, orange juice, vinegar, tarragon, and rosemary.

2. Add raw chicken breasts to marinade; cover and refrigerate 3–4 hours. Turn pieces of chicken to cover with marinade.

3. Heat grill to medium-high; place chicken on grill. Grill approximately 7–10 minutes on each side, until chicken is cooked through.

Herbed Chicken and Brown Rice Dinner

NUTRITIONAL ANALYSIS (per serving):

Calories: 300   Protein: 33g   Carbohydrates: 26g   Fat: 6g   Saturated Fat: 1g   Cholesterol: 75mg
Sodium: 112mg   Fiber: 0g   PCF Ratio: 45-36-19   Exchange Approx.: 1½ Starches, 2 Very-Lean Meats, 2 Lean Meats

INGREDIENTS | SERVES 4

1 tablespoon canola oil

4 (4-ounce) boneless chicken breast pieces, skin removed

¾ teaspoon garlic powder

¾ teaspoon dried rosemary

1 (10.5-ounce) can low-fat, reduced-sodium chicken broth

⅓ cup water

2 cups uncooked instant brown rice

1. Heat oil in large nonstick skillet on medium-high. Add chicken; sprinkle with ½ of garlic powder and crushed rosemary. Cover, and cook 4 minutes on each side, or until cooked through. Remove chicken from skillet and set aside.

2. Add broth and water to skillet; stir to deglaze pan and bring to a boil. Stir in rice and remaining garlic powder and rosemary. Top with chicken and cover; cook on low heat 5 minutes. Remove from heat and let stand, covered, 5 minutes.

Walnut Chicken with Plum Sauce

NUTRITIONAL ANALYSIS (per serving):

Calories: 159   Protein: 18g   Carbohydrates: 1g   Fat: 9g   Saturated Fat: 1g   Cholesterol: 44mg
Sodium: 51mg   Fiber: 1g   PCF Ratio: 47-3-51   Exchange Approx.: 2 Very-Lean Meats, 1½ Fats

INGREDIENTS | SERVES 4

¾ pound (12 ounces) raw boneless, skinless chicken breast

1 teaspoon sherry

1 egg white

2 teaspoons peanut oil

2 drops toasted sesame oil (optional)

⅓ cup ground walnuts

1. Preheat oven to 350°F. Cut chicken into bite-sized pieces; sprinkle with sherry and set aside.

2. In a small bowl, beat egg white and oils until frothy. Fold chicken pieces into egg mixture; roll individually in chopped walnuts.

3. Arrange chicken pieces on baking sheet treated with nonstick cooking spray. Bake 10–15 minutes, or until walnuts are lightly browned and chicken juices run clear. (Walnuts make the fat ratio of this dish high, so serve it with steamed vegetables and rice to bring the ratios into balance.)

Easy Chicken Paprikash

NUTRITIONAL ANALYSIS (per serving, using equal amounts of light and dark meat chicken):

Calories: 376   Protein: 22g   Carbohydrates: 58g   Fat: 6g   Saturated Fat: 2g
Cholesterol: 78mg   Sodium: 135mg   Fiber: 4g   PCF Ratio: 23-62-15
Exchange Approx.: ½ Very Lean Meat, ½ Lean Meat, 2½ Starches, 1 Vegetable, 1 Skim Milk

INGREDIENTS | SERVES 4

1 recipe Condensed Cream of Chicken Soup (Chapter 8)

½ cup skim milk

2 teaspoons paprika

⅛ teaspoon ground red pepper (optional)

¼ pound (4 ounces) chopped cooked boneless, skinless chicken

1½ cups sliced steamed mushrooms

½ cup diced steamed onion

½ cup nonfat plain yogurt

4 cups cooked medium-sized egg noodles

1. In saucepan, combine soup, skim milk, paprika, and pepper (if using); whisk until well mixed. Bring to a boil over medium heat, stirring occasionally.

2. Reduce heat to low and stir in chicken, mushrooms, and onion; cook until chicken and vegetables are heated through, about 10 minutes. Stir in yogurt.

3. To serve, put 1 cup of warm, cooked noodles on each of 4 plates. Top each portion with an equal amount of chicken mixture. Garnish by sprinkling with additional paprika, if desired.

For Best Results . . .

Mock condensed soup recipes are used in the dishes in this book so that you know the accurate Nutritional Analysis information. In all cases, you can substitute commercial canned condensed soups; however, be sure to use the lower fat and sodium varieties.

Chicken and Broccoli Casserole

NUTRITIONAL ANALYSIS (per serving):

Calories: 328   Protein: 26g   Carbohydrates: 20g   Fat: 17g   Saturated Fat: 6g
Cholesterol: 67mg   Sodium: 254mg   Fiber: 3g   PCF Ratio: 31-24-45
Exchange Approx.: 1 Very-Lean Meat, 1 Lean Meat, ½ High-Fat Meat, 1 Fat, 1 Vegetable, 1 Skim Milk, ½ Starch

INGREDIENTS | SERVES 4

2 cups broccoli

½ pound (8 ounces) cooked chopped chicken

½ cup skim milk

⅛ cup (2 tablespoons) real mayonnaise

¼ teaspoon curry powder

1 recipe Condensed Cream of Chicken Soup (Chapter 8)

1 tablespoon lemon juice

½ cup (2 ounces) grated Cheddar cheese

½ cup bread crumbs

1 teaspoon melted butter

1 teaspoon olive oil

1. Preheat oven to 350°F. Treat 11" × 7" casserole dish with nonstick spray.

2. Steam broccoli until tender; drain.

3. Spread out chicken on bottom of dish; cover with steamed broccoli.

4. In medium bowl, combine milk, mayonnaise, curry powder, soup, and lemon juice; pour over broccoli.

5. In small bowl, mix together cheese, bread crumbs, butter, and oil; sprinkle over top of casserole. Bake 30 minutes.

Chicken and Green Bean Stovetop Casserole

NUTRITIONAL ANALYSIS (per serving):

Calories: 305   Protein: 23g   Carbohydrates: 36g   Fat: 8g   Saturated Fat: 2g   Cholesterol: 48mg   Sodium: 101mg
Fiber: 6g   PCF Ratio: 30-46-24   Exchange Approx.: 1 Very-Lean Meat, 1 Lean Meat, 1 Vegetable, 1 Starch, 1 Skim Milk

INGREDIENTS | SERVES 4

1 recipe Condensed Cream of Chicken Soup (Chapter 8)

¼ cup skim milk

2 teaspoons Worcestershire sauce (recipe for homemade in Chapter 16)

1 teaspoon real mayonnaise

½ teaspoon onion powder

¼ teaspoon garlic powder

¼ teaspoon ground black pepper

1 (4-ounce) can sliced water chestnuts, drained

2½ cups frozen green beans, thawed

1 cup sliced mushrooms, steamed

½ pound (8 ounces) cooked chopped chicken

1⅓ cups cooked brown long-grain rice

1. Combine soup, milk, Worcestershire, mayonnaise, onion powder, garlic powder, and pepper in a saucepan; bring to a boil.

2. Reduce heat; add water chestnuts, green beans, mushrooms, and chicken. Simmer until vegetables and chicken are heated through, about 10 minutes. Serve over rice.

Veggie Filler

Steamed mushrooms are a low-calorie way to add flavor to a dish and "stretch" the meat. If you don't like mushrooms, you can substitute an equal amount of other low-calorie steamed vegetables like red and green peppers and not significantly affect the total calories in a recipe.

Chicken and Asparagus in White Wine Sauce

NUTRITIONAL ANALYSIS (per serving):

Calories: 186   Protein: 21g   Carbohydrates: 7g   Fat: 8g   Saturated Fat: 2g   Cholesterol: 51mg
Sodium: 57mg   Fiber: 2g   PCF Ratio: 46-16-38   Exchange Approx.: 2½ Very-Lean Meats, 1½ Vegetables, 1 Fat

INGREDIENTS | SERVES 4

4 boneless, skinless chicken breast halves
½ tablespoon butter
1 tablespoon olive oil
1 teaspoon garlic, finely chopped
½ cup onion, finely chopped
10 ounces asparagus spears, cut diagonally in 2" pieces
½ pound mushrooms
¼ cup dry white wine
¼ cup water
1 tablespoon parsley, chopped

1. Pound chicken pieces to ¼" thickness.

2. Melt butter and olive oil in a large skillet over medium heat. Add chopped garlic and onions; sauté 1–2 minutes.

3. Add chicken; cook 5 minutes, or until the chicken is brown on both sides. Remove chicken and set aside.

4. Add asparagus and mushrooms to skillet; cook 2–3 minutes.

5. Return chicken to skillet; add white wine and water. Bring to a quick boil; boil 2 minutes to reduce the liquid.

6. Reduce heat; cover and simmer 3 minutes, or until chicken and vegetables are tender. Add chopped parsley, salt and pepper to taste, and serve.

Chicken Kalamata

NUTRITIONAL ANALYSIS (per serving):

Calories: 311   Protein: 31g   Carbohydrates: 25g   Fat: 11g   Saturated Fat: 2g   Cholesterol: 66mg
Sodium: 787mg   Fiber: 6g   PCF Ratio: 38-31-31   Exchange Approx.: 4 Lean Meats, 2 Vegetables, 1 Starch, 2 Fats

INGREDIENTS | SERVES 4

2 tablespoons olive oil

1 cup onion, chopped

1 teaspoon garlic, minced

1½ cups green peppers, chopped

1 pound boneless, skinless chicken breast, cut into 4 pieces

2 cups tomatoes, diced

1 teaspoon oregano

½ cup pitted kalamata olives, chopped

1. Heat olive oil over medium heat in large skillet. Add onions, garlic, and peppers; sauté for about 5 minutes until onions are translucent.

2. Add chicken pieces; cook for about 5 minutes each side until lightly brown.

3. Add tomatoes and oregano. Reduce heat and simmer 20 minutes.

4. Add olives; simmer an additional 10 minutes before serving.

Are Olives Counted as a Fruit or Vegetable?

The short answer is: Neither! Even though olives are a fruit that grows on trees, their flesh is filled with a significant amount of oil and therefore is counted as a fat. Nine black olives or ten green olives equals 1 Fat Serving. The health benefits of olives (and olive oil) comes from the monounsaturated fats they contain. Olives are usually cured in a brine, salt, or olive oil, so if you must watch your salt intake, be careful how many you eat.

Chicken Breasts in Balsamic Vinegar Sauce

NUTRITIONAL ANALYSIS (per serving):

Calories: 200   Protein: 28g   Carbohydrates: 2g   Fat: 8g   Saturated Fat: 3g   Cholesterol: 73mg
Sodium: 381mg   Fiber: 0g   PCF Ratio: 58-4-38   Exchange Approx.: 4 Lean Meats, 1½ Fats

INGREDIENTS | SERVES 4

1 pound boneless, skinless chicken breasts, cut into 4 pieces

Pinch salt

¼ teaspoon pepper

1 tablespoon butter

1 tablespoon olive oil

¼ cup red onion, chopped

2 teaspoons garlic, finely chopped

3 tablespoons balsamic vinegar

1½ cups low-sodium chicken broth

1 teaspoon oregano

1. Sprinkle chicken with salt and pepper.

2. Heat butter and olive oil in large skillet over medium heat. Add chicken; cook until browned, about 5 minutes each side. Reduce heat and cook 12 minutes. Transfer to platter; cover and keep warm.

3. Add red onions and garlic to skillet; sauté over medium heat 3 minutes, scraping up browned bits. Add balsamic vinegar; bring to a boil. Boil 3 minutes, or until reduced to a glaze, stirring constantly.

4. Add chicken stock; boil until reduced to about ¾ cup liquid. Remove sauce from heat; add chopped oregano. Spoon sauce over chicken and serve immediately.

Chicken Thighs Cacciatore

NUTRITIONAL ANALYSIS (per serving):

Calories: 370   Protein: 19g   Carbohydrates: 48g   Fat: 9g   Saturated Fat: 2g   Cholesterol: 39mg
Sodium: 166mg   Fiber: 4g   PCF Ratio: 21-55-24   Exchange Approx.: 1½ Lean Meats, 2½ Starches, 1 Fat, 1 Vegetable

INGREDIENTS | SERVES 4

2 teaspoons olive oil

½ cup chopped onion

2 cloves garlic, minced

4 chicken thighs, skin removed

½ cup dry red wine

1 (14½-ounce) can unsalted diced tomatoes, undrained

1 teaspoon dried parsley

½ teaspoon dried oregano

¼ teaspoon pepper

⅛ teaspoon sugar

¼ cup grated Parmesan cheese

4 cups cooked spaghetti

2 teaspoons extra-virgin olive oil

1. Heat deep, nonstick skillet over medium-high heat; add 2 teaspoons olive oil. Add onion; sauté until transparent. Add garlic and chicken thighs; sauté 3 minutes on each side, or until lightly browned.

2. Remove thighs from pan; add wine, tomatoes and juices, parsley, oregano, pepper, and sugar. Stir well, bring to a boil. Add chicken back to pan; sprinkle Parmesan cheese over top. Cover, reduce heat, and simmer 10 minutes. Uncover and simmer 10 more minutes.

3. To serve, put 1 cup of cooked pasta on each of 4 plates. Top each serving with a chicken thigh; divide sauce between dishes. Drizzle ½ teaspoon extra-virgin olive oil over top of each dish and serve.

For Cheese Lovers!

Indulge your love of extra cheese and still have a main dish that's under 400 calories. Prepare Chicken Thighs Cacciatore according to recipe instructions. Top each portion with 1 tablespoon freshly grated Parmesan cheese. With cheese, analysis is: Calories: 398.22; Protein: 21.39g; Carbohydrates: 48.43g; Fat: 11.15g; Saturated Fat: 3.62g; Cholesterol: 43.87mg; Sodium: 282.14mg; Fiber: 3.81g; PCF Ratio: 23-51-26; Exchange Approx.: 2 Lean Meats, 2½ Starches, 1 Fat, 1 Vegetable.

Chicken with Portobello Mushrooms and Roasted Garlic

NUTRITIONAL ANALYSIS (per serving):

Calories: 335   Protein: 26g   Carbohydrates: 39g   Fat: 10g   Saturated Fat: 4g   Cholesterol: 56mg
Sodium: 261mg   Fiber: 3g   PCF Ratio: 30-45-25   Exchange Approx.: 2½ Lean Meats, ½ Fat, 8 Vegetables

INGREDIENTS | SERVES 4

1 tablespoon olive oil

4 boneless, skinless chicken breasts

1 cup reduced-sodium chicken broth

1 bulb garlic, dry roasted (see sidebar) and mashed into paste

1 tablespoon butter

2 cups Portobello mushrooms, chopped

½ teaspoon thyme

2 tablespoons feta cheese, crumbled

Dry-Roasted Garlic

To dry-roast garlic: Preheat oven to 350°F; lightly spray small, covered baking dish with nonstick spray. Slice off ½" from top of each garlic head; rub off any loose skins, being careful not to separate cloves. Place in baking dish, cut-side up (if roasting more than 1 head, arrange in dish so they don't touch). Cover and bake until the garlic cloves are very tender when pierced, about 30–45 minutes. Roasted garlic heads will keep in refrigerator 2–3 days.

1. Heat olive oil in large nonstick skillet; brown chicken breasts on both sides over medium heat, about 5 minutes per side. Add chicken broth and roasted garlic paste to pan; cover and simmer on low 10 minutes.

2. Meanwhile, sauté mushrooms and thyme in butter in separate, smaller saucepan. Simmer 2 minutes.

3. Add the mushrooms and thyme mixture to the chicken and simmer for an additional 2 minutes.

4. When serving, top each chicken breast with 1½ teaspoons feta cheese and pour sauce over the top.

Chipotle Chicken Wrap

NUTRITIONAL ANALYSIS (per serving):

Calories: 284   Protein: 24g   Carbohydrates: 28g   Fat: 8g   Saturated Fat: 2g   Cholesterol: 40mg
Sodium: 415mg   Fiber: 2g   PCF Ratio: 35-41-25   Exchange Approx.: 2 Starches, ½ Vegetable, 3 Lean Meats

INGREDIENTS | SERVES 4

12 ounces boneless, skinless chicken breast

1 tablespoon lime juice

1 tablespoon olive oil

1 teaspoon chipotle seasoning

⅛ teaspoon fresh ground pepper

4 whole-wheat tortillas

½ cup jar salsa

1 cup lettuce, chopped

1. Cut chicken into ½" strips. Place chicken, lime juice, olive oil, chipotle seasoning, and pepper in dish; mix well. Cover and allow chicken to marinate 1 hour.

2. Heat outdoor grill. Wrap tortillas in aluminum foil and place on top rack. Cook 7–9 minutes until done, turning strips once during cooking.

3. When ready to make wraps, place chicken strips in center of each heated tortilla, add 2 tablespoons salsa to each, top with chopped lettuce, and wrap.

What Is Chipotle?

A chipotle (chee-POTE-lay) is a smoke-dried jalapeño chili used in Mexican or Tex-Mex dishes. You can purchase dried chipotle peppers or a seasoning mix with chipotle peppers added. Mrs. Dash has a Southwest Chipotle Seasoning blend that is salt free!

Stovetop Grilled Turkey Breast

NUTRITIONAL ANALYSIS (per serving):

Calories: 207   Protein: 31g   Carbohydrates: 2g   Fat: 8g   Saturated Fat: 2g   Cholesterol: 85mg
Sodium: 68mg   Fiber: 0g   PCF Ratio: 62-3-35   Exchange Approx.: 4 Very-Lean Meats, ½ Fat

INGREDIENTS | SERVES 4

1 teaspoon cider vinegar

1 teaspoon garlic powder

1 teaspoon Dijon mustard

1 teaspoon brown sugar

¼ teaspoon black pepper

2 teaspoons olive oil

4 (4-ounce) turkey breast cutlets

Tip

Cutlets prepared this way tend to cook faster than on an outdoor grill. If using an indoor grill that cooks both sides at once, allow 4–5 minutes total cooking time. You can also use a well seasoned cast-iron skillet instead of a grill pan; however, you may need to introduce more oil to the pan to prevent the cutlets from sticking. Cooking time will be the same as with a grill pan. Be sure to adjust the Fat Exchange, if necessary.

1. In a medium bowl, combine vinegar, garlic powder, mustard, brown sugar, and black pepper; slowly whisk in olive oil to thoroughly combine and make a thin paste.

2. Rinse turkey cutlets and dry thoroughly on paper towels. If necessary to ensure a uniform thickness, put between sheets of plastic wrap and pound to flatten.

3. Pour paste into heavy-duty freezer-style resealable plastic bag. Add cutlets, moving around in mixture to coat all sides. Seal bag, carefully squeezing out as much air as possible. Refrigerate to allow turkey to marinate at least 1 hour, or as long as overnight.

4. Place nonstick hard-anodized stovetop grill pan over high heat. When pan is heated thoroughly, add cutlets. Lower heat to medium-high; cook cutlets 3 minutes on 1 side. Use tongs to turn; cook another 3 minutes, or until juices run clean.

Turkey Mushroom Burgers

NUTRITIONAL ANALYSIS (per serving):

Calories: 100   Protein: 15g   Carbohydrates: 3g   Fat: 3g   Saturated Fat: 1g   Cholesterol: 34mg
Sodium: 36mg   Fiber: 1g   PCF Ratio: 60-10-30   Exchange Approx.: 1 Lean Meat, 1 Vegetable, ½ Fat

INGREDIENTS | YIELDS 8 LARGE BURGERS

1-pound turkey breast

1 pound fresh button mushrooms

1 tablespoon olive oil

1 teaspoon butter

1 clove garlic, minced

1 tablespoon green onion, chopped

¼ teaspoon dried thyme

¼ teaspoon dried oregano

¼ teaspoon freshly ground black pepper

Cayenne pepper or dried red pepper flakes, to taste (optional)

1. Cut turkey into even pieces about 1" square. Place cubes in freezer 10 minutes, or long enough to allow turkey to become somewhat firm.

2. In a covered microwave-safe container, microwave mushrooms on high 3–4 minutes, or until they begin to soften and sweat. Set aside to cool slightly.

3. Process turkey in food processor until ground, scraping down sides of bowl as necessary. Add oil, butter, garlic, onion, and mushrooms (and any resulting liquid from the mushrooms); process until mushrooms are ground, scraping down sides of bowl as necessary. Add remaining ingredients; pulse until mixed. Shape into 8 equal-sized patties. Cooking times will vary according to method used and how thick burgers are.

Turkey Marsala with Fresh Peas

NUTRITIONAL ANALYSIS (per serving):

Calories: 278   Protein: 30g   Carbohydrates: 14g   Fat: 7g   Saturated Fat: 3g   Cholesterol: 78mg
Sodium: 208mg   Fiber: 2g   PCF Ratio: 50-24-27   Exchange Approx.: 4 Very-Lean Meats, ½ Starch, ½ Vegetable, 1 Fat

INGREDIENTS | SERVES 4

¼ cup all-purpose flour

¼ teaspoon salt

¼ teaspoon pepper

½ teaspoon paprika

1 pound raw turkey breast cutlets, sliced ¼" thick

1 tablespoon olive oil

1 tablespoon butter

½ cup onion, thinly sliced

½ cup Marsala wine

½ cup fresh or frozen peas

Quick Tip

It's easy to prepare quick and healthy meals if you keep skinless, boneless chicken or turkey in the freezer. If you use an indoor grill, you don't even need to thaw them first. You can prepare a quick sauce or glaze in the time it takes for the chicken or turkey to cook.

1. In a plastic zip-top bag, mix together flour, salt, pepper, and paprika. Place turkey cutlets in plastic bag; shake to coat cutlets with flour.

2. Heat olive and butter in large skillet; sauté onions for about 5 minutes, until browned.

3. Add coated turkey cutlets; brown on both sides, approximately 7–8 minutes on each side.

4. Add Marsala to pan; stir well to combine. Bring to a boil; reduce heat. Turn cutlets to coat both sides.

5. Add peas; continue to cook, stirring, another 2–3 minutes. Serve.

Spicy Grilled Turkey Burgers

NUTRITIONAL ANALYSIS (per serving):

Calories: 176   Protein: 26g   Carbohydrates: 5g   Fat: 5g   Saturated Fat: 2g   Cholesterol: 125mg
Sodium: 155mg   Fiber: 0g   PCF Ratio: 63-12-25   Exchange Approx.: 3½ Very-Lean Meats, 1 Fat

---

INGREDIENTS | SERVES 4

1 pound ground turkey

¼ cup bread crumbs

1 tablespoon Cajun-blend seasoning
(Chapter 17) or commercial salt-free blend

1 egg

1 tablespoon fresh cilantro, finely
chopped

2 teaspoons jalapeño pepper, minced

Nonstick cooking spray

1. Combine all ingredients well; shape into 4 patties.

2. Spray grill with nonstick cooking spray. Grill burgers approximately 6 minutes on each side, or until cooked through.

Proper Poultry and Meat Handling

Be sure to wash any utensil that comes in contact with raw poultry in hot, soapy water and rinse well. This includes washing any utensil each time it's used to baste grilling, roasting, or baking poultry.

Turkey Chili

NUTRITIONAL ANALYSIS (per serving):

Calories: 281   Protein: 26g   Carbohydrates: 38g   Fat: 4g   Saturated Fat: 1g   Cholesterol: 49mg   Sodium: 347mg
Fiber: 11g   PCF Ratio: 35-52-13   Exchange Approx.: 2 Starches, 2 Vegetables, 3 Very-Lean Meats, 1½ Fats

INGREDIENTS | SERVES 6

1 pound ground turkey

1 cup onions, chopped

½ cup green pepper, chopped

2 teaspoons garlic, finely chopped

2 (28-ounce) cans crushed canned tomatoes

1 cup canned black beans, drained

1 cup canned red kidney beans, drained

3 tablespoons chili powder

1 tablespoon ground cumin

1 teaspoon crushed red pepper

Dash Tabasco

1. Brown ground turkey in large nonstick pot over medium-high heat.

2. Drain off any fat; add chopped onion, green pepper, and garlic. Continue cooking until onion is translucent, about 5 minutes.

3. Add remaining ingredients; bring to a slow boil.

4. Reduce heat, cover, and let simmer at least 2–3 hours before serving.

Honey and Cider Glaze for Baked Chicken

NUTRITIONAL ANALYSIS (per serving, glaze only):

Calories: 10 Protein: 0g Carbohydrates: 2g Fat: 0g Saturated Fat: 0g Cholesterol: 0mg Sodium: 55mg
Fiber: 0g PCF Ratio: 9-90-1 Exchange Approx.: 1 Free Condiment

INGREDIENTS | SERVES 4

3 tablespoons cider or apple juice

½ teaspoon honey

1 teaspoon lemon juice

1 teaspoon Bragg's Liquid Aminos

½ teaspoon lemon zest

Spice Tea Chicken Marinade

Steep 4 orange or lemon spice tea bags in 2 cups boiling water for 4 minutes. Dissolve 1 teaspoon honey into the tea, pour it over 4 chicken pieces, and marinate for 30 minutes. Occasionally turn and baste any exposed portions of chicken. Pour the tea into the roasting pan to provide moisture—discard it after cooking.

1 Preheat oven to 375°F. Combine all ingredients in microwave-safe bowl; microwave on high 30 seconds. Stir until honey is dissolved.

2. To use glaze, arrange 4 boneless chicken pieces with skin removed on rack placed in roasting pan or broiling pan. Brush or spoon 1 teaspoon of glaze over top of each piece. Baste halfway through cooking time, and again 5 minutes before chicken is done. Allow chicken to sit 5 minutes before serving.

Turkey Kielbasa with Red Beans and Rice

NUTRITIONAL ANALYSIS (per serving):

Calories: 297   Protein: 15g   Carbohydrates: 41g   Fat: 9g   Saturated Fat: 3g   Cholesterol: 32mg   Sodium: 679mg
Fiber: 7g   PCF Ratio: 19-54-26   Exchange Approx.: 2 Starches, 1½ Vegetables, 1 Lean Meat, 1 Very-Lean Meat, 3 Fats

INGREDIENTS | SERVES 5

2 cups canned pinto beans, drained and rinsed

2 cups canned diced tomatoes

½ cup water

1 cup onion, diced

2 teaspoons Cajun-blend seasoning (Chapter 17)

8 ounces turkey kielbasa sausage, cut into 1" pieces

½ cup brown rice

1½ cups water

1. Combine pinto beans, canned tomatoes, water, onion, Cajun seasoning, and kielbasa in slow cooker; set on low and cook 4–6 hours.

2. In separate saucepan, bring brown rice and 1½ cups water to boil; reduce heat and simmer on low heat 35–40 minutes.

3. Serve beans and sausage over rice.

CHAPTER 11

Fish and Seafood Dishes

Fish Stock

NUTRITIONAL ANALYSIS (per serving):

Calories: 40   Protein: 5g   Carbohydrates: 0g   Fat: 2g   Saturated Fat: 1g   Cholesterol: 2mg
Sodium: Variable   Fiber: 0g   PCF Ratio: 55-0-45   Exchange Approx.: 1 Very-Lean Meat

**INGREDIENTS | YIELDS 4 CUPS;
SERVING SIZE: 1 CUP**

4 cups fish heads, bones, and trimmings
(approx. 1 pound)
2 stalks celery and leaves, chopped
1 onion, chopped
1 carrot, peeled and chopped
1 bay leaf
4 sprigs fresh parsley
Sea salt and pepper, to taste (optional)

Tip
To make stock from shellfish, simply substitute shrimp, crab, or lobster shells for the fish heads and bones.

1. Use your own fish trimmings (saved in bag in the freezer) or ask the butcher at your local fish market or supermarket for fish trimmings. Wash the trimmings well.

2. In a stockpot, combine all ingredients; add enough water to cover everything by an inch or so. Bring to a boil over high heat; reduce heat to low. Skim off foam that rises to top. Cover and simmer 20 minutes.

3. Remove from heat; strain through a sieve, discarding all solids. Refrigerate or freeze.

Asian-Style Fish Cakes

NUTRITIONAL ANALYSIS (per serving):

Calories: 66   Protein: 11g   Carbohydrates: 1g   Fat: 2g   Saturated Fat: 1g   Cholesterol: 41mg
Sodium: 112mg   Fiber: 0mg   PCF Ratio: 69-8-23   Exchange Approx.: 1 Lean Meat, 1 Free Condiment

INGREDIENTS | SERVES 8

1-pound catfish fillet

2 green onions, minced

1 banana pepper, cored, seeded, and chopped

2 cloves garlic, minced

1 tablespoon ginger, grated or minced

1 tablespoon Bragg's Liquid Aminos

1 tablespoon lemon juice

1 teaspoon lemon zest

Old Bay Seasoning, optional (Chapter 17)

Tip

For crunchy fish cakes, coat each side in rice flour and then lightly spritz the tops of the patties with olive or peanut oil before baking as directed.

1. Preheat oven to 375°F. Cut fish into 1" pieces. Combine with green onions, banana pepper, garlic, ginger, Bragg's Liquid Aminos, lemon juice, and lemon zest in food processor; process until chopped and mixed. (You do not want to purée this mixture; it should be a rough chop.) Add Old Bay seasoning, if using; stir to mix.

2. Form fish mixture into patties of about 2 tablespoons each; you should have 16 patties total. Place patties on baking sheet treated with nonstick cooking spray; bake 12–15 minutes, or until crisp. (Alternatively, you can fry these in a nonstick pan about 4 minutes on each side.)

Salmon Patties

NUTRITIONAL ANALYSIS (per serving):

Calories: 168   Protein: 17g   Carbohydrates: 3g   Fat: 9g   Saturated Fat: 2g   Cholesterol: 70mg
Sodium: 92mg   Fiber: 0g   PCF Ratio: 42-8-50   Exchange Approx.: 2 Lean Meats, ½ Fat, ½ Starch

INGREDIENTS | SERVES 5

2 cups flaked cooked salmon (no salt added)

6 soda crackers, crushed

1 egg

½ cup skim milk

1 small onion, chopped

1 tablespoon fresh parsley, chopped

1 tablespoon unbleached all-purpose flour

1 tablespoon olive oil

Ener-G rice flour (optional)

1. Place salmon in a bowl; flake with fork. Add crushed crackers, egg, milk, onion, parsley, and flour; mix well. Gently form 5 patties.

2. Heat oil in nonstick skillet over medium heat. (Optional: Lightly dust patties with some Ener-G rice flour for crispier patties.) Fry on both sides until browned, about 5 minutes per side.

Crab Cakes with Sesame Crust

NUTRITIONAL ANALYSIS (per serving):

Calories: 108 Protein: 9g Carbohydrates: 3g Fat: 6g Saturated Fat: 1g Cholesterol: 45mg
Sodium: 171mg Fiber: 1g PCF Ratio: 34-11-55 Exchange Approx.: 1 Very-Lean Meat, 1½ Fats

INGREDIENTS | SERVES 5

1 pound (16 ounces) lump crabmeat
1 egg
1 tablespoon fresh ginger, minced
1 small scallion, finely chopped
1 tablespoon dry sherry
1 tablespoon freshly squeezed lemon juice
6 tablespoons real mayonnaise
Sea salt and freshly ground white pepper, to taste (optional)
Old Bay seasoning, to taste (optional)
¼ cup lightly toasted sesame seeds

1. Preheat oven to 375°F. In large bowl, mix together crab, egg, ginger, scallion, sherry, lemon juice, mayonnaise, and seasonings, if using.

2. Form the mixture into 10 equal cakes. Spread sesame seeds over sheet pan; dip both sides of cakes to coat them. Arrange cakes on baking sheet treated with nonstick spray. Typical baking time is 8–10 minutes, depending on thickness of cakes.

Barley-Spinach-Fish Bake

NUTRITIONAL ANALYSIS (per serving):

Calories: 239   Protein: 26g   Carbohydrates: 15g   Fat: 8g   Saturated Fat: 1g   Cholesterol: 67mg
Sodium: 418mg   Fiber: 3g   PCF Ratio: 44-26-30   Exchange Approx.: 3 Lean Meats, ½ Starch, 1 Vegetable, 1½ Fats

INGREDIENTS | SERVES 4

½ tablespoon olive oil
¼ cup scallions, chopped
1 clove garlic, minced
¼ teaspoon rosemary
¼ teaspoon marjoram
¼ teaspoon salt
1 cup pearl barley, cooked
5 ounces (½ box) frozen chopped spinach, thawed and drained
¼ cup sundried tomatoes, chopped
4 (12-inch) squares of aluminum foil
4 (4-ounce) fish fillets
3 tablespoons white wine
Salt and fresh ground pepper, to taste

Cooking barley

Pearl barley takes longer to cook than quick-cooking barley, so you will want to prepare it in advance. To prepare: bring ½ cup pearl barley and 1 cup water to a boil. Reduce heat, cover, and simmer for 35–45 minutes, or until all water is absorbed. Pearl barley makes a good side dish on its own with the addition of spices or vegetables.

1. Preheat oven to 400°F (or outdoor grill can be used).

2. Heat oil in medium nonstick skillet; add scallions and sauté 2 minutes. Add garlic, rosemary, marjoram, and salt; continue to cook another 3 minutes, until scallions are tender. Add cooked barley, spinach, and sundried tomatoes; mix well.

3. Place aluminum foil squares on work surface; place a fish fillet in center of each square. Divide barley mixture equally; place on top of each fillet. Sprinkle with white wine, salt, and pepper.

4. Fold aluminum foil loosely to enclose filling. Place packets on baking sheet (or directly on grill if using outdoor grill); bake 15 minutes, or until fish is tender and flakes easily.

Grilled Salmon with Roasted Peppers

NUTRITIONAL ANALYSIS (per serving):

Calories: 269   Protein: 24g   Carbohydrates: 8g   Fat: 16g   Saturated Fat: 3g   Cholesterol: 67mg
Sodium: 321mg   Fiber: 1g   PCF Ratio: 36-11-53   Exchange Approx.: 3½ Lean Meats, 1 Vegetable, 1 Fat

INGREDIENTS | SERVES 4

4 (4-ounce) salmon steaks
1 tablespoon reduced-sodium soy sauce
1 tablespoon brown sugar
1 tablespoon olive oil
2 large red bell peppers
1 tablespoon balsamic vinegar
½ teaspoon dried thyme
¼ teaspoon fresh-ground pepper

Wasabi Marinade

Wasabi, also known as Japanese horserad-ish, can be purchased in raw form or as a powder or paste. It adds a hot, pungent flavor to fish and works especially well with salmon. To make a marinade for salmon or other fish, mix 1 teaspoon wasabi powder (or paste) with 2 tablespoons low-sodium soy sauce, ½ teaspoon grated ginger, and 1 teaspoon sesame oil. Coat fish with the marinade and grill.

1. Place salmon in shallow dish. Mix together soy sauce, brown sugar, and olive oil; pour over salmon and cover both sides with marinade. Set aside.

2. Prepare roasted red peppers following procedure in Chapter 16. Once peppers are roasted and peeled, cut into strips and sprinkle balsamic vinegar, thyme, and pepper. Set aside.

3. Heat grill. Remove salmon from the marinade; grill over medium heat approximately 8 minutes on one side. Turn and grill on other side until salmon is cooked and tender, about 4–5 minutes longer. Remove from heat.

4. Top each salmon steak with marinated roasted red peppers.

Baked Bread Crumb–Crusted Fish with Lemon

NUTRITIONAL ANALYSIS (per serving, without salt):

Calories: 137 Protein: 24g Carbohydrates: 5g Fat: 3g Saturated Fat: 1g Cholesterol: 36mg Sodium: 73mg
Fiber: 2g PCF Ratio: 68-14-18 Exchange Approx.: 2 Very-Lean Meats, ½ Starch, ½ Free Condiment

INGREDIENTS | SERVES 6

2 large lemons
¼ cup dried bread crumbs
1½ pounds (24 ounces) halibut fillets
Sea or kosher salt and freshly ground white or black pepper, to taste (optional)

Lemon Infusion

Mildly flavored fish such as catfish, cod, halibut, orange roughy, rockfish, and snapper benefit from the distinctive flavor of lemon. Adding slices of lemon to top of fish allows the flavor to infuse into fish.

1. Preheat oven to 375°F. Wash 1 lemon; cut into thin slices. Grate 1 tablespoon of zest from the second lemon, then juice it. Combine grated zest and bread crumbs in small bowl; stir to mix. Set aside.

2. Put lemon juice in shallow dish; arrange lemon slices in bottom of baking dish treated with nonstick spray. Dip fish pieces in lemon juice; set on lemon slices in baking dish.

3. Sprinkle bread crumb mixture evenly over fish pieces along with salt and pepper, if using; bake until crumbs are lightly browned and fish is just opaque, 10–15 minutes. (Baking time will depend on thickness of fish.) Serve immediately, using lemon slices as garnish.

Baked Red Snapper Almandine

NUTRITIONAL ANALYSIS (per serving, without salt):

Calories: 178   Protein: 24g   Carbohydrates: 3g   Fat: 7g   Saturated Fat: 2g   Cholesterol: 47mg
Sodium: 73mg   Fiber: 1g   PCF Ratio: 56-7-37   Exchange Approx.: 3 Lean Meats

INGREDIENTS | SERVES 4

1 pound (16 ounces) red snapper fillets

Sea or kosher salt and freshly ground white or black pepper, to taste (optional)

4 teaspoons all-purpose flour

2 teaspoons olive oil

2 tablespoons ground raw almonds

2 teaspoons unsalted butter

1 tablespoon lemon juice

1. Preheat oven to 375°F. Rinse red snapper fillets and dry between layers of paper towels. Season with salt and pepper, if using; sprinkle with flour, front and back.

2. In an ovenproof nonstick skillet, sauté fillets in olive oil until nicely browned on both sides, about 5 minutes per side.

3. Combine ground almonds and butter in microwave-safe dish. Microwave on high 30 seconds, or until butter is melted; stir to combine. Pour almond-butter mixture and lemon juice over fillets; bake 3–5 minutes, or until almonds are nicely browned.

A-Taste-of-Italy Baked Fish

NUTRITIONAL ANALYSIS (per serving):

Calories: 128   Protein: 22g   Carbohydrates: 7g   Fat: 1g   Saturated Fat: 0g   Cholesterol: 50mg
Sodium: 312mg   Fiber: 1g   PCF Ratio: 68-23-9   Exchange Approx.: 2½ Very-Lean Meats, 1½ Vegetables

INGREDIENTS | SERVES 4

1 pound (16 ounces) cod fillets

1 (14½-ounce) can stewed tomatoes

¼ teaspoon dried minced onion

½ teaspoon dried minced garlic

¼ teaspoon dried basil

¼ teaspoon dried parsley

⅛ teaspoon dried oregano

⅛ teaspoon sugar

1 tablespoon grated Parmesan cheese

1. Preheat oven to 375°F. Rinse cod with cold water and pat dry with paper towels.

2. In 2–3-quart baking pan or casserole treated with nonstick cooking spray, combine all ingredients except fish; mix.

3. Arrange fillets over mixture, folding thin tail ends under; spoon mixture over fillets. For fillets about 1" thick, bake uncovered 20–25 minutes, or until fish is opaque and flaky.

Crunchy "Fried" Catfish Fillets

NUTRITIONAL ANALYSIS (per serving, without salt):

Calories: 244   Protein: 21g   Carbohydrates: 18g   Fat: 9g   Saturated Fat: 2g   Cholesterol: 53mg
Sodium: 248mg   Fiber: 1g   PCF Ratio: 35-30-35   Exchange Approx.: 3 Lean Meats, 1 Starch

---

INGREDIENTS | SERVES 4

1 egg white (from a large egg), room temperature

¼ cup bread crumbs

¼ cup enriched white cornmeal

1 teaspoon grated lemon zest

½ teaspoon crushed dried basil

¼ cup all-purpose flour

⅛ teaspoon kosher or sea salt (optional)

¼ teaspoon lemon pepper

Zesty Crunch

Grated lemon or lime zest is a great way to give added citrus flavor to a crunchy bread-crumb topping for fish.

1. Preheat oven to 450°F; treat shallow baking pan with nonstick spray. Rinse catfish and dry between layers of paper towels.

2. In shallow dish, beat egg white until frothy. In another dish, combine bread crumbs, cornmeal, lemon zest, and basil. In third dish, combine flour, salt (if using), and lemon pepper.

3. Dip fish into flour mixture to coat 1 side of each fillet. Shake off any excess flour mixture, then dip flour-covered side of fillet into egg white. Next, coat covered side of fillet with bread-crumb mixture.

4. Arrange prepared fillets side by side, coated-sides up, on prepared baking pan. Tuck in any thin edges. Bake 6–12 minutes, or until fish flakes easily with a fork.

Jon's Fish Tacos

NUTRITIONAL ANALYSIS (per serving):

Calories: 383   Protein: 29g   Carbohydrates: 40g   Fat: 12g   Saturated Fat: 2g   Cholesterol: 60mg   Sodium: 400mg
Fiber: 4g   PCF Ratio: 30-42-28   Exchange Approx.: 3½ Very-Lean Meats, 2 Starches, 1 Vegetable, 1 Fat

INGREDIENTS | SERVES 4

¼ cup light mayonnaise
½ cup plain nonfat yogurt
¼ cup onion, chopped
2 tablespoons jalapeño pepper, minced
2 teaspoons cilantro, minced
2 cups cabbage, shredded
¼ cup lime juice
1 clove garlic, minced
1 tablespoon canola oil
1 pound tilapia fillets
4 whole-wheat tortillas, 6" diameter
Aluminum foil
Nonstick cooking spray
1 cup tomato, chopped

1. In medium bowl, whisk together mayonnaise, yogurt, onion, jalapeño, and cilantro. Stir in shredded cabbage; chill.

2. In separate bowl, combine lime juice, garlic, and canola oil to make a marinade for fish. Pour over fish; cover and refrigerate at least 1 hour.

3. Place fish on aluminum-lined grill (spray aluminum with cooking spray); cook 6–7 minutes on each side, until fish is tender and beginning to flake.

4. While fish is cooking, loosely wrap whole-wheat tortilla in large piece of aluminum foil to heat.

5. To assemble tacos, cut fish into strips; divide into 4 portions. Place strips in center of each heated tortilla. Top with coleslaw mixture and chopped tomatoes. Add fresh ground pepper, if desired.

Sweet Onion–Baked Yellowtail Snapper

NUTRITIONAL ANALYSIS (per serving, no salt):

Calories: 189   Protein: 25g   Carbohydrates: 13g   Fat: 4g   Saturated Fat: 1g   Cholesterol: 42mg   Sodium: 77mg
Fiber: 1g   PCF Ratio: 53-28-19   Exchange Approx.: 1 Lean Meat, 2 Very-Lean Meats, 1 Vegetable, ½ Starch

INGREDIENTS | SERVES 4

2 cups sliced Vidalia onions

1 tablespoon balsamic vinegar

2 teaspoons brown sugar

4 teaspoons olive oil

1 pound (16 ounces) skinless yellowtail snapper fillets

Sea salt and freshly ground white or black pepper, to taste (optional)

1. In covered microwave-safe dish, microwave onion on high 5 minutes, or until transparent. Carefully remove cover; stir in vinegar and brown sugar. Cover; allow to sit several minutes so onion absorbs flavors.

2. Heat a nonstick pan on medium-high; add olive oil. Transfer steamed onion mixture to pan; sauté until browned but not crisp. (Be careful, as onions will burn easily because of brown sugar; if onion browns too quickly, lower heat and add a few tablespoons of water.) Cook until all liquid has evaporated from pan, stirring often. Onions should have a shiny and dark caramelized color. (This can be prepared 2–3 days in advance; store tightly covered in refrigerator.)

3. Preheat oven to 375°F. Rinse snapper in cold water and dry between paper towels. Arrange on baking sheet treated with nonstick spray. Spoon caramelized onions over tops of fillets, pressing to form a light crust over top of fish. Bake 12–15 minutes, or until fish flakes easily with a fork. Serve immediately with Madeira sauce divided on 4 plates with fish placed on top.

Stir-Fried Ginger Scallops with Vegetables

NUTRITIONAL ANALYSIS (per serving):

Calories: 145 Protein: 22g Carbohydrates: 8g Fat: 3g Saturated Fat: 1g Cholesterol: 37mg
Sodium: 373mg Fiber: 2g PCF Ratio: 61-23-16 Exchange Approx.: 3 Very-Lean Meats, ½ Vegetable

INGREDIENTS | SERVES 4

1 pound (16 ounces) scallops

1 teaspoon peanut or sesame oil

1 tablespoon chopped fresh ginger

2 cloves garlic, minced

4 scallions, thinly sliced (optional)

1 teaspoon rice wine vinegar

2 teaspoons Bragg's Liquid Aminos

½ cup low-fat reduced-sodium chicken broth

2 cups broccoli florets

1 teaspoon cornstarch

¼ teaspoon toasted sesame oil

1. Rinse scallops and pat dry between layers of paper towels. If necessary, slice scallops so they're uniform size. Set aside.

2. Add peanut oil to heated nonstick deep skillet or wok; sauté ginger, garlic, and scallions if using, 1–2 minutes, being careful ginger doesn't burn. Add vinegar, Liquid Aminos, and broth; bring to a boil. Remove from heat.

3. Place broccoli in large, covered microwave-safe dish; pour chicken broth mixture over top. Microwave on high 3–5 minutes, depending on preference. (Keep in mind that vegetables will continue to steam for a minute or so if cover remains on dish.)

4. Heat skillet or wok over medium-high temperature. Add scallops; sauté 1 minute on each side. (Do scallops in batches if necessary; be careful not to overcook.) Remove scallops from pan when done; set aside. Drain (but do not discard) liquid from broccoli; return liquid to bowl and transfer broccoli to heated skillet or wok. Stir-fry vegetables to bring up to serving temperature.

5. Meanwhile, in small cup or bowl, add enough water to cornstarch to make a slurry or roux. Whisk slurry into reserved broccoli liquid; microwave on high 1 minute. Add toasted sesame oil; whisk again. Pour thickened broth mixture over broccoli; toss to mix. Add scallops back to broccoli mixture; stir-fry over medium heat to return scallops to serving temperature. Serve over rice or pasta; adjust Exchange Approximations accordingly.

Scallops and Shrimp with White Bean Sauce

NUTRITIONAL ANALYSIS (per serving):

Calories: 231   Protein: 27g   Carbohydrates: 18g   Fat: 4g   Saturated Fat: 1g   Cholesterol: 105mg
Sodium: 217mg   Fiber: 7g   PCF Ratio: 49-34-17   Exchange Approx.: 3 Very-Lean Meats, ½ Fat, 1 Starch, ½ Vegetable

INGREDIENTS | SERVES 4

½ cup finely chopped onion, steamed

2 cloves garlic, minced

2 teaspoons olive oil, divided

¼ cup dry white wine

¼ cup tightly packed fresh parsley leaves

¼ cup tightly packed fresh basil leaves

1⅓ cups canned cannellini (white) beans, drained and rinsed

¼ cup low-fat, reduced-sodium chicken broth

½ pound (8 ounces) shrimp, shelled and deveined

½ pound (8 ounces) scallops

1. In nonstick saucepan, sauté onion and garlic in 1 teaspoon of oil over moderately low heat, for about 5 minutes until onion is soft. Add wine; simmer until wine is reduced by ½. Add parsley, basil, ⅓ cup of beans, and chicken broth; simmer, stirring constantly, 1 minute.

2. Transfer bean mixture to blender or food processor; purée. Pour purée back into saucepan; add remaining beans; simmer 2 minutes.

3. In nonstick skillet, heat remaining 1 teaspoon of oil over moderately high heat until it is hot but not smoking. Sauté shrimp 2 minutes on each side, or until cooked through. Using slotted spoon, transfer shrimp to plate; cover to keep warm. Add scallops to skillet; sauté 1 minute on each side, or until cooked through. To serve, divide bean sauce between 4 shallow bowls and arrange shellfish over top.

Pasta and Smoked Trout with Lemon Pesto

NUTRITIONAL ANALYSIS (per serving):

Calories: 209   Protein: 10g   Carbohydrates: 23g   Fat: 8g   Saturated Fat: 1g   Cholesterol: 4mg   Sodium: 151mg
Fiber: 1g   PCF Ratio: 20-45-36   Exchange Approx.: 1 Fat, 1½ Lean Meats, 1 Carbohydrate/Starch

INGREDIENTS | SERVES 4

2 cloves garlic

2 cups fresh basil leaves, tightly packed

⅛ cup pine nuts, toasted

2 teaspoons fresh lemon juice

2 teaspoons water

4 teaspoons extra-virgin olive oil

4 tablespoons grated Parmesan cheese, divided

1⅓ cups uncooked linguini or other pasta (to yield 2 cups cooked pasta)

2 ounces whole boneless smoked trout

Freshly ground black pepper, to taste

1. Put garlic in food processor; pulse until finely chopped. Add basil, pine nuts, lemon juice, and water; process until just puréed. (Note: You can substitute fresh parsley for basil; supplement flavor by adding some dried basil, too, if you do.) Add olive oil and 3 tablespoons of Parmesan cheese; pulse until pesto is smooth, occasionally scraping down side of bowl, if necessary. Set aside.

2. Cook pasta according to package directions. While it is cooking, flake trout. When pasta is cooked, pulse pesto to ensure it has remained blended; toss pesto and trout with pasta. Sprinkle remaining Parmesan and some pepper on top of each serving. (Although this recipe uses heart-healthy extra-virgin olive oil, it is a little higher in fat, but still low in calories. Consult your dietitian if you have any question whether you should include this recipe in your meal plans.)

Grilled Haddock with Peach-Mango Salsa

NUTRITIONAL ANALYSIS (per serving, including ½ cup peach-mango salsa):

Calories: 204   Protein: 22g   Carbohydrates: 11g   Fat: 8g   Saturated Fat: 1g   Cholesterol: 65mg
Sodium: 467mg   Fiber: 2g   PCF Ratio: 43-22-35   Exchange Approx.: 3 Very-Lean Meats, 1 Fat, ½ Fruit

INGREDIENTS | SERVES 4

2 tablespoons olive oil
2 tablespoons lime juice
¼ teaspoon salt
¼ teaspoon ground pepper
1 pound haddock fillets
Fresh Peach-Mango Salsa (Chapter 16)

1. Mix olive oil, lime juice, salt, and pepper in a shallow dish; add haddock. Turn and coat fish with marinade.

2. Heat gas grill or broiler. Spray large piece of aluminum foil with nonstick cooking spray. Place fillets on foil; cook 7–8 minutes on each side, or until fish is tender when pierced with a fork.

3. Top each piece of fish with ½ cup Fresh Peach-Mango Salsa.

Sesame Shrimp and Asparagus

NUTRITIONAL ANALYSIS (per serving):

Calories: 257   Protein: 28g   Carbohydrates: 23g   Fat: 6g   Saturated Fat: 1g   Cholesterol: 172mg
Sodium: 173mg   Fiber: 3g   PCF Ratio: 44-35-21   Exchange Approx.: 3 Very-Lean Meats, ½ Vegetable, 1 Starch

INGREDIENTS | SERVES 4

2 teaspoons canola oil

2 cloves garlic, chopped

1 tablespoon fresh ginger root, grated

1 pound medium shrimp

2 tablespoons dry white wine

½ pound asparagus, cut diagonally into 1" pieces

2 cups whole-grain pasta, cooked

½ teaspoon sesame seeds

¼ cup scallions, thinly sliced

1 teaspoon sesame oil

1. Heat canola oil in wok or large nonstick skillet. Stir fry garlic, ginger root, and shrimp over high heat until shrimp begins to turn pink, about 2 minutes.

2. Add white wine and asparagus; stir fry an additional 3–5 minutes.

3. Add pasta, sesame seeds, scallions, and sesame oil; toss lightly and serve.

Spicy "Fried" Fish Fillet

NUTRITIONAL ANALYSIS (per serving):

Calories: 230   Protein: 24g   Carbohydrates: 9g   Fat: 10g   Saturated Fat: 2g   Cholesterol: 116mg
Sodium: 412mg   Fiber: 1g   PCF Ratio: 44-17-39   Exchange Approx.: 3 Very-Lean Meats, 2 Fats, ½ Starch

INGREDIENTS | SERVES 4

⅓ cup cornmeal

½ teaspoon salt

1 teaspoon chipotle seasoning

1 egg

2 tablespoons 1% milk

16 ounces flounder, cut into 4 pieces

2 tablespoons olive oil

1. Combine cornmeal, salt, and chipotle seasoning in shallow dish.

2. Beat egg and milk together in shallow dish.

3. Dip fish in egg mixture; coat each fillet with cornmeal mixture.

4. Heat olive oil in nonstick skillet; brown fillets until golden and crispy, about 6–7 minutes each side.

Fresh Tomato and Clam Sauce with Whole-Grain Linguini

NUTRITIONAL ANALYSIS (per serving):

Calories: 361   Protein: 13g   Carbohydrates: 60g   Fat: 8g   Saturated Fat: 1g   Cholesterol: 7mg   Sodium: 356mg
Fiber: 8g   PCF Ratio: 14-66-20   Exchange Approx.: 2½ Starches, 1½ Very-Lean Meats, 3 Vegetables, 1½ Fats

INGREDIENTS | SERVES 4

3 dozen (36) littleneck clams

2 tablespoons olive oil

5 cloves garlic, chopped

½ cup red bell pepper, chopped

4 cups fresh tomatoes, peeled and chopped

3 tablespoons fresh parsley, chopped

1 tablespoon fresh basil, chopped

¼ teaspoon salt

¼ teaspoon red pepper flakes

½ teaspoon oregano

½ cup dry white wine

8 ounces whole-grain linguini

Tip

This recipe works well with canned clams if you are unable to get fresh. Canned clams are quite high in sodium, which will need to be taken into consideration. If using canned clams, you will need 1 (8-ounce) can of minced clams and 1 (10-ounce) can of whole clams. Reserve the clam juice and add to the sauce.

1. Before preparing this dish (preferably several hours or more), place clams in bowl of cold water with handful of cornmeal added; keep refrigerated. (This will help purge clams of any sand or other debris.) When ready to cook, rinse and scrub clams.

2. Heat olive oil, garlic, and red pepper in a deep skillet. Add chopped tomatoes, parsley, basil, salt, red pepper flakes, and oregano, bring to quick boil, then reduce heat and simmer 15–20 minutes.

3. Stir in white wine; add clams on top of tomato sauce. Cover and steam until clams open.

4. Meanwhile, boil water and cook pasta to al dente.

5. Serve tomato sauce and clams over pasta.

CHAPTER 12

Casseroles and Stews

Condensed Cream of Mushroom Soup

NUTRITIONAL ANALYSIS (per recipe):

Calories: 92   Protein: 3g   Carbohydrates: 21g   Fat: 1g   Saturated Fat: 0g   Cholesterol: 0mg   Sodium: 13mg
Fiber: 3g   PCF Ratio: 12-84-4   Exchange Approx.: Will depend on serving size and preparation method

**INGREDIENTS | YIELDS EQUIVALENT OF
1 (10.75-OUNCE) CAN**

¾ cup finely chopped fresh mushrooms

½ cup water

⅛ cup Ener-G potato flour

Optional ingredients:

1 teaspoon chopped onion

1 tablespoon chopped celery

½ cup water

⅛ cup Ener-G potato flour

Potato Flour Substitute?

Instant mashed potatoes can replace potato flour; however, the amount needed will vary according to the brand of potatoes. Also, you'll need to consider other factors such as added fats and hydrogenated oils.

1. In a microwave-safe covered container, microwave mushrooms (and onion and celery, if using) for 2 minutes, or until tender. (About ¾ cup chopped mushrooms will yield ½ cup steamed ones.) Reserve any resulting liquid; add enough water to equal 1 cup.

2. Place all ingredients in a blender; process. The thickness of soup concentrate will vary according to how much moisture remains in mushrooms. If necessary, add 1–2 tablespoons of water to achieve a paste. (Low-sodium canned mushrooms work in this recipe, but the Nutritional Analysis assumes fresh mushrooms are used. Adjust sodium content accordingly.)

Condensed Cream of Chicken Soup

NUTRITIONAL ANALYSIS (per recipe):

Calories: 158   Protein: 4g   Carbohydrates: 35g   Fat: 1g   Saturated Fat: 0g   Cholesterol: 1mg   Sodium: 162mg
Fiber: 2g   PCF Ratio: 9-88-3   Exchange Approx.: Will depend on serving size and preparation method

**INGREDIENTS | YIELDS EQUIVALENT OF
1 (10.75-OUNCE) CAN**

1 cup water

¾ teaspoon Minor's Low-Sodium
Chicken Base

¼ cup Ener-G potato flour

Place all ingredients in blender; process until well blended.

Condensed Cream of Chicken Soup with Regular Chicken Broth

For the equivalent of 1 (10.75-ounce) can of condensed chicken soup, blend 1 cup reduced-fat canned chicken broth with ¼ cup Ener-G potato flour. Will last, refrigerated, 3 days. Nutritional Analysis: Calories: 181.20; Protein: 7.61g; Carbohydrates: 34.14g; Fat: 1.50g; Saturated Fat: 0.42g; Cholesterol: 0.00mg; Sodium: 785.20mg; Fiber: 2.36g; PCF Ratio: 17-76-7; Exchange Approx.: will depend on serving size and preparation method.

Condensed Cream of Celery Soup

NUTRITIONAL ANALYSIS (per recipe):

Calories: 85   Protein: 2g   Carbohydrates: 20g   Fat: 0g   Saturated Fat: 0g   Cholesterol: 0mg   Sodium: 79mg
Fiber: 2g   PCF Ratio: 9-89-2   Exchange Approx.: Will depend on serving size and preparation method

INGREDIENTS | YIELDS EQUIVALENT OF 1 (10.75-OUNCE) CAN

½ cup steamed chopped celery
½ cup water
⅛ cup Ener-G potato flour

1. In a microwave-safe, covered container, microwave celery for 2 minutes, or until tender. Do not drain any resulting liquid. If necessary, add enough water to bring celery and liquid to 1 cup total.

2. Place all ingredients in blender; process. Use immediately, or store in a covered container in refrigerator for use within 3 days. Thickness of concentrate will depend on how much moisture remains in celery; add 1–2 tablespoons of water, if necessary, to achieve a paste.

Condensed Cream of Potato Soup

NUTRITIONAL ANALYSIS (per recipe):

Calories: 103   Protein: 2g   Carbohydrates: 24g   Fat: 0g   Saturated Fat: 0g   Cholesterol: 0mg   Sodium: 9mg
Fiber: 2g   PCF Ratio: 8-91-1   Exchange Approx.: Will depend on serving size and preparation method

**INGREDIENTS | YIELDS EQUIVALENT OF
1 (10.75-OUNCE) CAN**

½ cup peeled, diced potatoes

½ cup water

1 tablespoon Ener-G potato flour

Tip

The Nutritional Analysis for this recipe assumes you'll use the entire tablespoon of Ener-G potato flour; however, the amount needed will depend on the amount of starch in the potatoes you use. For example, new potatoes will require more Ener-G potato flour than larger, Idaho-style potatoes.

1. Place potatoes and water in covered microwave-safe bowl; microwave on high for 4–5 minutes, until potatoes are fork-tender.

2. Pour potatoes and water in blender, being careful of steam. Remove vent from blender lid; process until smooth. Add Ener-G flour 1 teaspoon at a time while blender is running.

Condensed Tomato Soup

NUTRITIONAL ANALYSIS (per serving):

Calories: 136   Protein: 4g   Carbohydrates: 31g   Fat: 1g   Saturated Fat: 0g   Cholesterol: 0mg   Sodium: 352mg
Fiber: 4g   PCF Ratio: 11-83-6   Exchange Approx.: Will depend on serving size and preparation method

INGREDIENTS | YIELDS EQUIVALENT OF 1 (10.75-OUNCE) CAN

1 cup peeled chopped tomato, with juice

Additional tomato juices (if necessary)

¼ teaspoon baking soda

⅛ cup Ener-G potato flour

Direct Preparation

If you'll be making the soup immediately after you prepare the condensed soup recipe, you can simply add your choice of the additional 1 cup of liquid (such as skim milk, soy milk, or water) to the blender and use that method to mix the milk and soup concentrate together. Pour the combined mixture into your pan or microwave-safe dish.

1. Place tomato in microwave-safe bowl; microwave on high for 2–3 minutes, until tomato is cooked. Add additional tomato juices if necessary to bring mixture back up to 1 cup.

2. Add baking soda; stir vigorously until bubbling stops.

3. Pour cooked tomato mixture into blender; add potato flour, 1 tablespoon at a time, processing until well blended.

Condensed Cheese Soup

NUTRITIONAL ANALYSIS (per recipe):

Calories: 315   Protein: 20g   Carbohydrates: 18g   Fat: 18g   Saturated Fat: 11g   Cholesterol: 56mg   Sodium: 384mg
Fiber: 1g   PCF Ratio: 26-23-51   Exchange Approx.: Will depend on serving size and preparation method

INGREDIENTS | YIELDS EQUIVALENT OF 1 (10.75-OUNCE) CAN

½ cup water

⅛ cup Ener-G potato flour

¼ cup nonfat cottage cheese

2 ounces American, Cheddar, or Colby Cheese, shredded (to yield ½ cup)

Place water, potato flour, and cottage cheese in blender; process until well blended. Stir in shredded cheese. Cheese will melt as casserole is baked, prepared in microwave, or cooked on stovetop, according to recipe instructions.

Be Aware of Your Exchanges

When using any soup preparation method, you'll need to add the appropriate Exchange Approximations for each serving amount (usually ¼ of the total) of whatever condensed soup you make. For example, broth-based soups like chicken and cream of mushroom or celery would be a Free Exchange; cream of potato soup would add 1 Carbohydrate/Starch.

Soup Preparation Method

NUTRITIONAL ANALYSIS (per serving, skim milk):

Additional Calories: 21   Protein: 2g   Carbohydrates: 3g   Fat: 0g   Saturated Fat: 0g   Cholesterol: 1mg   Sodium: 32mg
Fiber: 0g   PCF Ratio: 39-56-5   Exchange Approx.: 1 Low-Fat Milk for entire pot of soup; divide accordingly per serving

INGREDIENTS | SERVES 4

Any previous condensed soup recipe
1 cup skim milk

To use any of the homemade condensed soup recipes as soup, add 1 cup of skim milk (or soy milk or water) to a pan. Stir using a spoon or whisk to blend. Cook over medium heat for 10 minutes until mixture begins to simmer. Season according to taste.

Traditional Stovetop Tuna-Noodle Casserole

NUTRITIONAL ANALYSIS (per serving):

Calories: 245 Protein: 20g Carbohydrates: 33g Fat: 4g Saturated Fat: 2g Cholesterol: 46mg
Sodium: 241mg Fiber: 4g PCF Ratio: 32-53-15 Exchange Approx.: 1½ Starches, 1 Vegetable, 1 Medium-Fat Meat

INGREDIENTS | SERVES 4

1⅓ cups egg noodles (yields 2 cups when cooked)

1 recipe Condensed Cream of Mushroom Soup (Chapter 8)

1 teaspoon steamed chopped onion

1 tablespoon steamed chopped celery

½ cup skim milk

1 ounce American, Cheddar, or Colby cheese, shredded (to yield ¼ cup)

1 cup frozen mixed peas and carrots

1 cup steamed sliced fresh mushrooms

1 can water-packed tuna, drained

1. Cook egg noodles according to package directions. Drain and return to pan.

2. Add all remaining ingredients to pan; stir to blend. Cook over medium heat, stirring occasionally, until cheese is melted. (The Nutritional Analysis for this recipe assumes egg noodles were cooked without salt.)

Extra-Rich Stovetop Tuna-Noodle Casserole

Add 1 medium egg (beaten) and 1 table-spoon mayonnaise to give casserole taste of rich, homemade egg noodles, while still maintaining good fat ratio. It's still less than 300 calories per serving, too! Nutritional Analysis: Calories: 275; Protein: 21g; Carbohydrates: 34g; Fat: 7g; Saturated Fat: 2g; Cholesterol: 94mg; Sodium: 281mg; Fiber: 4g; PCF Ratio: 30-48-21; Exchange Approx.: 1½ Breads, 1 Vegetable, 1 Meat, 1 Medium-Fat Meat.

Chicken and Mushroom Rice Casserole

NUTRITIONAL ANALYSIS (per serving):

Calories: 165   Protein: 9g   Carbohydrates: 30g   Fat: 1g   Saturated Fat: 0g   Cholesterol: 15mg
Sodium: 41mg   Fiber: 3g   PCF Ratio: 23-71-6   Exchange Approx.: 1 Very Lean Meat, 1 Starch, 1 Vegetable

INGREDIENTS | SERVES 8

1 recipe Condensed Cream of Chicken Soup (Chapter 8)

1 cup diced chicken breast

1 large onion, chopped

½ cup chopped celery

1 cup uncooked rice (not instant rice)

Freshly ground black pepper, to taste (optional)

1 teaspoon dried Herbes de Provence blend (Chapter 17), optional

2 cups boiling water

2½ cups chopped broccoli flowerets

1 cup sliced fresh mushrooms

1. Preheat oven to 350°F. In 4-quart casserole dish (large enough to prevent boilovers in oven) treated with nonstick spray, combine condensed soup, chicken breast, onion, celery, rice, and seasonings; mix well. Pour boiling water over top; bake, covered, 30 minutes.

2. Stir casserole; add broccoli and mushrooms. Replace cover; return to oven to bake additional 20–30 minutes, or until celery is tender and rice has absorbed all liquid.

Ham and Artichoke Hearts Scalloped Potatoes

NUTRITIONAL ANALYSIS (per serving, without salt):

Calories: 269   Protein: 21g   Carbohydrates: 31g   Fat: 8g   Saturated Fat: 4g   Cholesterol: 28mg   Sodium: 762mg
Fiber: 6g   PCF Ratio: 31-44-25   Exchange Approx.: 1½ Lean Meats, ½ High-Fat Meat, 1½ Vegetables, 1 Starch

INGREDIENTS | SERVES 4

2 cups frozen artichoke hearts

1 cup chopped onion

4 small potatoes, thinly sliced

Sea salt and freshly ground black pepper, to taste (optional)

1 tablespoon lemon juice

1 tablespoon dry white wine

1 cup Mock Cream (Chapter 16)

½ cup nonfat cottage cheese

1 teaspoon dried parsley

1 teaspoon garlic powder

⅛ cup freshly grated Parmesan cheese

¼ pound (4 ounces) lean ham, cubed

2 ounces Cheddar cheese, grated (to yield ½ cup)

1. Preheat oven to 300°F.

2. Thaw artichoke hearts and pat dry with a paper towel. In deep casserole dish treated with nonstick spray, layer artichokes, onion, and potatoes; lightly sprinkle salt and pepper over top (if using).

3. In a food processor or blender, combine lemon juice, wine, Mock Cream, cottage cheese, parsley, garlic powder, and Parmesan cheese; process until smooth. Pour over layered vegetables; top with ham. Cover casserole dish (with a lid or foil); bake 35–40 minutes, or until potatoes are cooked through.

4. Remove cover; top with Cheddar cheese. Return to oven another 10 minutes, or until cheese is melted and bubbly. Let rest 10 minutes before cutting.

Simple Substitutions

Artichoke hearts can be expensive. You can substitute cabbage, broccoli, or cauliflower (or a mixture of all 3) for the artichokes.

Hearty Beef Stew (Fast and Slow Method)

NUTRITIONAL ANALYSIS (per serving):

Calories: 326 Protein: 26g Carbohydrates: 32g Fat: 10g Saturated Fat: 3g Cholesterol: 88mg
Sodium: 335mg Fiber: 4g PCF Ratio: 32-39-28 Exchange Approx.: 3 Lean Meats, 1 Starch, 3 Vegetables

INGREDIENTS | SERVES 4

1 tablespoon olive oil

12 ounces beef round, cut into 1" cubes

1 cup onion, chopped

2 cups potatoes, cut into 1" pieces

½ cup carrots, cut into 1" pieces

1 cup green beans

½ cup turnip, peeled and cut into 1" pieces

1 tablespoon parsley

¼ teaspoon Tabasco

1 cup low-sodium V-8 Juice

¼ teaspoon salt

1 tablespoon all-purpose flour

¼ cup water

1. Heat olive oil in pressure cooker and brown meat. Add onions, potatoes, carrots, green beans, turnip, parsley, Tabasco, V-8 juice, and salt.

2. Close cover securely; place pressure regulator on vent pipe and cook for 10–12 minutes with pressure regulator rocking slowly. (Or follow manufacturer instructions for your pressure cooker.) Cool down pressure cooker at once (nonelectric pressure cookers).

3. If desired, make paste of 1 tablespoon flour and ¼ cup water; stir into stew to thicken. Heat and stir liquid until thickened.

Slow-Cook Method for Beef Stew

If you don't have pressure cooker, you can make in slow cooker. First, heat olive oil in skillet. Dredge meat in 1–2 tablespoons flour; add to skillet and brown. Transfer to slow cooker; add onions, V-8, potatoes, carrots, green beans, turnip, salt, parsley, and Tabasco. Cook on low-medium for 4–6 hours.

Main Dish Pork and Beans

NUTRITIONAL ANALYSIS (per serving):

Calories: 153   Protein: 11g   Carbohydrates: 24g   Fat: 2g   Saturated Fat: 1g   Cholesterol: 18mg
Sodium: 146mg   Fiber: 5g   PCF Ratio: 29-61-10   Exchange Approx.: 2 Lean Meats, ½ Fruit/Misc. Carbohydrate

INGREDIENTS | SERVES 4

1⅓ cups cooked pinto beans

2 tablespoons ketchup

¼ teaspoon Dijon mustard

¼ teaspoon dry mustard

1 teaspoon cider vinegar

4 tablespoons diced red onion

1 tablespoon 100% maple syrup

1 teaspoon brown sugar

¼ pound (4 ounces) slow-cooked shredded pork

⅛ cup (2 tablespoons) apple juice or cider

Preheat oven to 350°F. In casserole dish treated with nonstick spray, combine beans, ketchup, Dijon mustard, dry mustard, vinegar, onion, syrup, and brown sugar. Layer meat over top of bean mixture. Pour apple juice or cider over pork. Bake for 20–30 minutes, or until mixture is well heated and bubbling. Stir well before serving.

Easy Oven Beef Burgundy

NUTRITIONAL ANALYSIS (per serving):

Calories: 266   Protein: 34g   Carbohydrates: 12g   Fat: 6g   Saturated Fat: 2g   Cholesterol: 82mg
Sodium: 388mg   Fiber: 2g   PCF Ratio: 56-20-23   Exchange Approx.: 4 Lean Meats, 2 Vegetables, 1 Fat

INGREDIENTS | SERVES 4

2 tablespoons all-purpose flour
1 pound beef round, cubed
2 tablespoons all-purpose flour
1 cup carrots, sliced
1 cup onions, chopped
1 cup celery, sliced
1 clove garlic, finely chopped
¼ teaspoon pepper
¼ teaspoon marjoram
¼ teaspoon thyme
½ teaspoon salt
2 tablespoons balsamic vinegar
½ cup dry red wine
½ cup water
1 cup fresh mushrooms, sliced

1. Preheat oven to 325°F.

2. Dredge meat cubes in flour; place in 3-quart covered baking dish or Dutch oven. Add carrots, onions, celery, garlic, pepper, marjoram, thyme, salt, and vinegar; combine.

3. Pour red wine and water over mixture. Cover and bake 1 hour.

4. Remove from oven; mix in mushrooms.

5. Return to oven for 1 hour, or until beef cubes are tender.

Shrimp Microwave Casserole

NUTRITIONAL ANALYSIS (per serving):

Calories: 196   Protein: 18g   Carbohydrates: 27g   Fat: 2g   Saturated Fat: 1g   Cholesterol: 131mg
Sodium: 290mg   Fiber: 2g   PCF Ratio: 35-56-9   Exchange Approx.: 1 Starch, 1 Vegetable, 1 Medium-Fat Meat

INGREDIENTS | SERVES 4

1⅓ cups uncooked egg noodles (to yield 4½ [½-cup] servings)

1 cup chopped green onion

1 cup chopped green pepper

1 cup sliced mushrooms

1 recipe Condensed Cream of Celery Soup (Chapter 8)

1 teaspoon Worcestershire sauce (see recipe for Homemade Worcestershire in Chapter 16)

4 drops Tabasco (optional)

¼ cup diced canned pimientos

½ cup pitted, chopped ripe olives

½ cup skimmed milk

½ pound (8 ounces) cooked, deveined, shelled shrimp

1. Cook egg noodles according to package directions; drain and keep warm.

2. Place green onion and green pepper in covered microwave-safe dish; microwave on high 1 minute. Add mushrooms; microwave another minute, or until all vegetables are tender.

3. Add soup, Worcestershire sauce, Tabasco (if using), pimiento, olives, and milk; stir well. Microwave, covered, 1–2 minutes, until mixture is hot and bubbly.

4. Add cooked shrimp and noodles; stir to mix. Microwave 30 seconds to 1 minute, or until mixture is hot.

Eggplant and Tomato Stew

NUTRITIONAL ANALYSIS (per serving):

Calories: 135 Protein: 4g Carbohydrates: 26g Fat: 3g Saturated Fat: 1g Cholesterol: 0mg
Sodium: 22mg Fiber: 9g PCF Ratio: 12-69-19 Exchange Approx.: ½ Fat, 4 Vegetables

INGREDIENTS | SERVES 4

2 eggplants, trimmed but left whole

2 teaspoons olive oil

1 medium-sized Spanish onion, chopped

1 teaspoon garlic, chopped

2 cups cooked or canned unsalted tomatoes, chopped, with liquid

Optional seasonings, to taste:

1 teaspoon hot pepper sauce

Ketchup

Nonfat plain yogurt

Fresh parsley sprigs

1. Preheat oven to 400°F.

2. Roast eggplants on baking sheet until soft, about 45 minutes. Remove all meat from eggplants.

3. In large sauté pan, heat oil; sauté onions and garlic. Add eggplant and all other ingredients, except yogurt and parsley. Remove from heat and transfer to food processor; pulse until it becomes creamy.

4. Serve at room temperature, garnished with a dollop of yogurt and parsley, if desired.

CHAPTER 13

Pasta, Rice, Grains, and Beans

Quick Tomato Sauce

NUTRITIONAL ANALYSIS (per serving, without salt):

Calories: 40   Protein: 1g   Carbohydrates: 6g   Fat: 2g   Saturated Fat: 0g   Cholesterol: 0mg   Sodium: 10mg
Fiber: 1g   PCF Ratio: 9-49-42   Exchange Approx.: 1 Vegetable, ½ Fat

---

INGREDIENTS | SERVES 8

2 pounds very ripe tomatoes

2 tablespoons extra-virgin olive oil

2 cloves garlic, minced

½ teaspoon ground cumin

2 large sprigs fresh thyme, or ½ teaspoon dried thyme

1 bay leaf

Kosher or sea salt and freshly ground black pepper, to taste (optional)

3 tablespoons total of chopped fresh basil, oregano, tarragon, and parsley or cilantro, or a combination of all the listed herbs, to taste. If using dried herbs, reduce the amount to 1 tablespoon

1. Peel and seed tomatoes; chop with knife or food processor.

2. Heat large skillet; add olive oil. Reduce heat to low; sauté garlic and cumin.

3. Add tomatoes, thyme, bay leaf, salt, and pepper, if using. If using dried herbs, add now. Simmer, uncovered, over medium heat for 8–10 minutes, stirring often; reduce heat to maintain a simmer, if necessary. Simmer until tomatoes are soft and sauce has thickened, about 30 minutes. Discard bay leaf and thyme sprigs; adjust seasoning to taste. If using fresh herbs, add just before serving.

Remember . . .

The addition of ¼ teaspoon granulated sugar in tomato sauce helps cut the acidity of the tomatoes without affecting the Exchange Approximations for the recipe.

Basic Tomato Sauce

NUTRITIONAL ANALYSIS (per serving, without salt):

Calories: 37 Protein: 1g Carbohydrates: 5g Fat: 2g Saturated Fat: 0g Cholesterol: 0mg Sodium: 9mg
Fiber: 1g PCF Ratio: 9-55-36 Exchange Approx.: 1½ Vegetables

**INGREDIENTS | YIELDS ABOUT 5 CUPS;
SERVING SIZE: ¼ CUP**

2 tablespoons olive oil

2 cups coarsely chopped yellow onion

½ cup sliced carrots

2 cloves garlic, minced

4 cups canned Italian plum tomatoes
with juice

1 teaspoon dried oregano

1 teaspoon dried basil

¼ teaspoon sugar

Kosher or sea salt and freshly ground
black pepper, to taste (optional)

Dash of ground anise seed (optional)

1. Heat olive oil in large, deep skillet or saucepan over medium-high heat. Add onions, carrots, and garlic; sauté until onions are transparent. (For a richer-tasting sauce, allow onions to caramelize or reach a light golden brown.)

2. Purée tomatoes in food processor.

3. Add the puréed tomatoes, oregano, basil, and sugar to onion mixture along with salt, pepper, and anise, if using. Simmer, partially covered, 45 minutes.

4. If you prefer a smoother sauce, process sauce in food processor again.

Culinary Antacids

Stir in 2 teaspoons Smucker's Low-Sugar Grape Jelly to tame hot chili or acidic sauces such as tomato sauce. You won't really notice the flavor of the jelly, and it will do a great job of reducing any tart, bitter, or acidic tastes in your sauce.

Fresh Garden Spaghetti Sauce

NUTRITIONAL ANALYSIS (per serving):

Calories: 154   Protein: 6g   Carbohydrates: 26g   Fat: 5g   Saturated Fat: 1g   Cholesterol: 0mg
Sodium: 867mg   Fiber: 6g   PCF Ratio: 15-61-25   Exchange Approx.: 5 Vegetables, 1 Fat

INGREDIENTS | SERVES 12

3 tablespoons olive oil

1 cup celery, chopped

1 cup onion, finely chopped

1 cup green (or sweet red) pepper, chopped

2 cloves garlic, crushed

8 cups fresh tomatoes, peeled and crushed

1 (5½-ounce) can tomato paste

1 cup zucchini, grated

1 tablespoon fresh oregano, chopped

1 tablespoon fresh basil, chopped

½ teaspoon crushed red pepper

½ cup dry red wine

1. In large, heavy sauce pan or Dutch oven, heat oil. Add celery, onion, and peppers; sauté 5 minutes. Add crushed garlic; sauté additional 2 minutes.

2. Add crushed tomatoes, tomato paste, zucchini, oregano, basil, and red pepper. Bring to a boil; reduce heat and simmer for 2–3 hours.

3. Add wine during last 30 minutes of cooking.

Tip

Don't waste unused tomato paste left in can. Spoon out tablespoon-sized portions and place on plastic wrap or in sandwich baggies. Seal packages and store in freezer. When you need tomato paste in a recipe, add frozen paste directly to sauce; no need to defrost.

Fusion Lo Mein

NUTRITIONAL ANALYSIS (per serving):

Calories: 126   Protein: 5g   Carbohydrates: 26g   Fat: 1g   Saturated Fat: 0g   Cholesterol: 0mg
Sodium: 35mg   Fiber: 4g   PCF Ratio: 14-77-9   Exchange Approx.: 1 Starch, 1 Vegetable, ½ Fruit

INGREDIENTS | SERVES 6

2 tablespoons rice vinegar

2 tablespoons thawed pineapple-orange juice

2 teaspoons minced shallots

2 teaspoons lemon juice

1 teaspoon cornstarch

1 teaspoon Worcestershire sauce (see recipe for homemade in Chapter 16)

1 teaspoon honey

2 cloves garlic, minced

1 teaspoon olive oil

¾ cup chopped green onions

1 cup diagonally sliced (¼" thick) carrots

1 cup julienned yellow bell pepper

1 cup julienned red bell pepper

3 cups small broccoli florets

1 cup fresh bean sprouts

1½ cups cooked pasta

1. In food processor or blender, combine vinegar, juice concentrate, shallots, lemon juice, cornstarch, Worcestershire, honey, and garlic; process until smooth.

2. Heat wok or large nonstick skillet coated with cooking spray over medium-high heat until hot; add olive oil. Add onions; stir-fry for 1 minute.

3. Add carrots, bell peppers, and broccoli; stir-fry another minute. Cover pan; cook for 2 more minutes.

4. Add vinegar mixture and sprouts. Bring mixture to a boil; cook, uncovered, 30 seconds, stirring constantly.

5. Add cooked pasta; toss to mix.

Roasted Butternut Squash Pasta

NUTRITIONAL ANALYSIS (per serving):

Calories: 216   Protein: 5g   Carbohydrates: 40g   Fat: 5g   Saturated Fat: 1g   Cholesterol: 0mg   Sodium: 8mg
Fiber: 2g   PCF Ratio: 9-70-21   Exchange Approx.: 2 Starches, 1 Fat, ½ Vegetable

INGREDIENTS | SERVES 4

1 butternut squash
4 teaspoons extra-virgin olive oil
1 clove garlic, minced
1 cup chopped red onion
2 teaspoons red wine vinegar
¼ teaspoon dried oregano
2 cups cooked pasta
Freshly ground black pepper (optional)

Tip

For added flavor, use roasted instead of raw garlic. Roasting garlic causes it to caramelize, adding a natural sweetness.

1. Preheat oven to 400°F. Cut squash in half and scoop out seeds. Using nonstick spray, coat 1 side of 2 pieces of heavy-duty foil large enough to wrap squash halves. Wrap squash in foil; place on a baking sheet. Bake for 1 hour, or until tender.

2. Scoop out baked squash flesh and discard rind; rough-chop. Add olive oil, garlic, and onion to nonstick skillet; sauté for about 5 minutes until onion is transparent. (Alternatively, put oil, garlic, and onion in covered microwave-safe dish; microwave on high for 2–3 minutes.)

3. Remove pan from heat; stir in vinegar and oregano. Add squash; stir to coat in onion mixture. Add pasta; toss to mix. Season with freshly ground black pepper, if desired.

Pasta with Artichokes

NUTRITIONAL ANALYSIS (per serving):

Calories: 308   Protein: 10g   Carbohydrates: 47g   Fat: 9g   Saturated Fat: 2g   Cholesterol: 2mg   Sodium: 87mg
Fiber: 3g   PCF Ratio: 13-60-27   Exchange Approx.: 1 Medium-Fat Meat, 2 Vegetables, 1 Starch, 2 Fats

INGREDIENTS | SERVES 4

1 (10-ounce) package frozen artichoke hearts

1¼ cups water

1 tablespoon lemon juice

4 teaspoons olive oil

2 cloves garlic, minced

¼ cup sundried tomatoes packed in oil, drained and chopped

¼ teaspoon red pepper flakes

2 teaspoons dried parsley

2 cups cooked pasta

¼ cup grated Parmesan cheese

Freshly ground black pepper, to taste (optional)

1. Cook artichokes in water and lemon juice according to package directions; drain, reserving ¼ cup of liquid. Cool artichokes; cut into quarters.

2. Heat olive oil in nonstick skillet over medium heat. Add garlic; sauté 1 minute. Reduce heat to low. Stir in artichokes and tomatoes; simmer for 1 minute. Stir in reserved artichoke liquid, red pepper, and parsley; simmer for 5 minutes.

3. Pour artichoke sauce over pasta in a large bowl; toss gently to coat. Sprinkle with cheese and top with pepper, if desired.

Tip

You can decrease amount of water to 3 tablespoons and add it with artichokes and lemon juice to covered microwave-safe dish. Microwave according to package directions; reserve all liquid. This results in stronger lemon flavor, which compensates for lack of salt in recipe.

Pasta with Creamed Clam Sauce

NUTRITIONAL ANALYSIS (per serving):

Calories: 226 Protein: 15g Carbohydrates: 24g Fat: 7g Saturated Fat: 2g Cholesterol: 25mg
Sodium: 209mg Fiber: 1g PCF Ratio: 27-43-30 Exchange Approx.: 1 Lean Meat, 1 Starch, 1 Fat, ½ Skim Milk

INGREDIENTS | SERVES 4

1 (6½-ounce) can chopped clams

4 teaspoons olive oil

1 clove garlic, minced

1 tablespoon dry white wine or dry vermouth

½ cup Mock Cream (Chapter 16)

¼ cup freshly grated Parmesan cheese

2 cups cooked pasta

Freshly ground black pepper, to taste (optional)

1. Drain clams; reserve juice. Heat olive oil in large nonstick skillet. Add garlic; sauté 1 minute; stir in clams and sauté another minute. With slotted spoon, transfer clams to a bowl; cover to keep warm.

2. Add wine and reserved clam juice to skillet; bring to a boil and reduce by half. Lower heat and add Mock Cream; and cook for about 2-3 minutes, being careful not to boil cream.

3. Stir in Parmesan cheese; continue to heat another minute, stirring constantly.

4. Add pasta; toss with sauce. Divide into 4 equal servings; serve immediately, topped with freshly ground pepper, if desired.

Whole-Grain Noodles with Caraway Cabbage

NUTRITIONAL ANALYSIS (per serving):

Calories: 169 Protein: 6g Carbohydrates: 27g Fat: 5g Saturated Fat: 1g Cholesterol: 0mg
Sodium: 250mg Fiber: 5g PCF Ratio: 14-60-26 Exchange Approx.: 1 Starch, 1 Vegetable, 1 Fat

---

INGREDIENTS | SERVES 6

2 tablespoons olive oil

½ cup onion, chopped

2 cups cabbage, coarsely chopped

1½ cups Brussels sprouts, trimmed and halved

2 teaspoons caraway seed

1½ cups low-sodium chicken broth

¼ teaspoon fresh ground pepper

¼ teaspoon salt

6 ounces whole-grain noodles

1. Heat olive oil in large saucepan; sauté onions for about 5 minutes until translucent.

2. Add cabbage and Brussels sprouts; cook over medium heat for 3 minutes.

3. Stir in caraway seed, broth, pepper, and salt; Cover and simmer for 5–8 minutes until vegetables are crisp-tender.

4. Cook noodles in boiling water until tender; drain.

5. Mix noodles and vegetables together in a large bowl; serve.

Tuscan Pasta Fagioli

NUTRITIONAL ANALYSIS (per serving):

Calories: 317   Protein: 15g   Carbohydrates: 54g   Fat: 6g   Saturated Fat: 1g   Cholesterol: 2mg
Sodium: 248mg   Fiber: 11g   PCF Ratio: 18-65-17   Exchange Approx.: 3 Starches, ½ Vegetable, 1 Fat

INGREDIENTS | SERVES 6

2 tablespoons olive oil

⅓ cup onion, chopped

3 cloves garlic, minced

½ pound tomatoes, peeled and chopped

5 cups low-sodium vegetable stock

¼ teaspoon freshly ground pepper

3 cups cannellini beans, rinsed and drained

2½ cups whole-grain pasta shells

2 tablespoons Parmesan cheese

1. Heat olive oil in large pot; gently cook onions and garlic until soft but not browned. Add tomatoes, vegetable stock, and pepper.

2. Purée 1½ cups of cannellini beans in food processor or blender; add to stock. Cover and simmer 20–30 minutes

3. While stock is simmering, cook pasta until al dente; drain. Add remaining beans and pasta to stock; heat through. Serve with Parmesan cheese.

Brown Rice and Vegetable Sauté

NUTRITIONAL ANALYSIS (per serving):

Calories: 154   Protein: 5g   Carbohydrates: 26g   Fat: 4g   Saturated Fat: 1g   Cholesterol: 0mg
Sodium: 352mg   Fiber: 3g   PCF Ratio: 12-64-24   Exchange Approx.: 1 Starch, 1½ Vegetables, 1 Fat

INGREDIENTS | SERVES 4

½ cup brown rice

1 cup water

1 tablespoon olive oil

½ cup onions, chopped

1 cup red bell peppers, chopped

1 teaspoon garlic, minced

4 ounces mushrooms, sliced

12-ounce package fresh bean sprouts

1 tablespoon reduced-sodium soy sauce

1 teaspoon fresh ginger, grated

1. Add rice to water, bring to boil. Reduce heat; cover and simmer for 35–40 minutes, until cooked.

2. In large nonstick skillet or wok, heat olive oil. Add onions, red pepper and garlic; cook until onion is translucent.

3. Add mushrooms, bean sprouts, and soy sauce; cook on low heat for 3 minutes.

4. Add rice and ginger; mix ingredients. Cook on low additional for an 2–3 minutes.

Squash and Bulgur Pilaf

NUTRITIONAL ANALYSIS (per serving):

Calories: 151   Protein: 5g   Carbohydrates: 22g   Fat: 6g   Saturated Fat: 1g   Cholesterol: 0mg
Sodium: 190mg   Fiber: 5g   PCF Ratio: 13-54-32   Exchange Approx.: 1 Starch, ½ Vegetable, 2 Fats

INGREDIENTS | SERVES 6

1 tablespoon olive oil

½ cup onions, chopped

1 teaspoon garlic, minced

1½ cups yellow summer squash, cut into ½" pieces

1 cup bulgur wheat

1 tablespoon olive oil

2 cups low-sodium chicken broth

½ teaspoon cinnamon

¼ cup dried currants

¼ cup walnuts, chopped

1. In large nonstick skillet, sauté onions, garlic, yellow squash, and bulgur wheat in olive oil until onions are tender, about 5 minutes.

2. Stir in chicken broth and cinnamon; heat to boiling. Reduce heat and simmer, covered, for 10 minutes.

3. Stir in currants; continue to simmer for an additional 15 minutes. Add walnuts just before serving.

Herbed Quinoa with Sundried Tomatoes

NUTRITIONAL ANALYSIS (per serving):

Calories: 119   Protein: 5g   Carbohydrates: 21g   Fat: 2g   Saturated Fat: 0g   Cholesterol: 0mg
Sodium: 193mg   Fiber: 2g   PCF Ratio: 17-71-12   Exchange Approx.: 1 Starch, ½ Very-Lean Meat, 2 Fat

---

INGREDIENTS | SERVES 6

½ tablespoon olive oil

¼ cup onion, chopped

1 clove garlic, minced

1 cup quinoa

2 cups low-sodium chicken broth

½ cup fresh mushrooms, sliced

6 sundried tomatoes, cut into ¼" pieces

1 teaspoon Italian-blend seasoning

Cooking Time for Quinoa

Quinoa takes no longer to cook than rice or pasta, usually about 15 minutes. You can tell quinoa is cooked when grains have turned from white to transparent and spiral-like germ has separated from seed.

1. In medium saucepan, heat olive oil; sauté onions and garlic.

2. Rinse quinoa in very fine mesh strainer before cooking. Add quinoa and broth to saucepan; bring to a boil for 2 minutes. Add mushrooms, sundried tomatoes, and Italian seasoning.

3. Reduce heat and cover. Cook 15 minutes, or until all water is absorbed.

Quinoa with Roasted Vegetables

NUTRITIONAL ANALYSIS (per serving):

Calories: 120   Protein: 4g   Carbohydrates: 9g   Fat: 4g   Saturated Fat: 0g   Cholesterol: 0mg
Sodium: 151mg   Fiber: 4g   PCF Ratio: 12-62-26   Exchange Approx.: 1 Starch, 1 Vegetable, 2 Fats

INGREDIENTS | SERVES 4

⅔ cup green pepper

½ cup red pepper (mildly hot variety)

3 cups eggplant, cut into 1" cubes

2 cloves garlic, finely chopped

1 tablespoon olive oil

½ teaspoon Texas Seasoning (Chapter 17)

¼ teaspoon cumin

½ cup quinoa

1 cup water

¼ teaspoon salt

Another Idea

Cook quinoa as outlined in steps 3 and 4. Combine with 3 cups of Oven-Roasted Ratatouille recipe found in Chapter 14. Nutritional Analysis for 1 cup serving: Calories: 162; Protein: 7g; Carbohydrates: 26g; Fat: 3g; Saturated Fat: 0g; Cholesterol: 1mg; Sodium: 202mg; Fiber: 4g; PCF Ratio: 13-69-18; Exchange Approx.: 1 Starch, 2 Vegetables, ½ Fat.

1. Preheat oven to 375°F. Combine peppers, eggplant, garlic, olive oil, Texas Seasoning, and cumin in 2-quart baking dish. Cover and roast for 20 minutes.

2. Remove cover; continue to roast in oven for about 30 minutes until vegetables are browned and cooked soft. Remove from oven; place cover.

3. Rinse quinoa in very fine mesh strainer before cooking. Bring water and salt to a boil; add quinoa and bring to a boil for 5 minutes. Cover; remove from heat and let stand 15 minutes.

4. Once quinoa is cooked and all water is absorbed, add roasted vegetables and serve.

Kasha-Stuffed Red Peppers

NUTRITIONAL ANALYSIS (per serving):

Calories: 383   Protein: 22g   Carbohydrates: 54g   Fat: 12g   Saturated Fat: 5g   Cholesterol: 40mg   Sodium: 387mg
Fiber: 11g   PCF Ratio: 22-53-25   Exchange Approx.: 2 Starches, 4 Vegetables, 1½ Lean Meats, 2 Fats

INGREDIENTS | SERVES 4

2 pounds red peppers (4 large)

1 cup kasha

1 egg white, lightly beaten

Nonstick cooking spray

2 cups low-sodium beef broth

4 ounces lean ground beef

1 cup onion, finely chopped

5 ounces (½ package) frozen chopped spinach, thawed and drained

½ cup feta cheese, crumbled

½ cup canned diced tomatoes

1 teaspoon oregano

⅛ teaspoon crushed red pepper

1½ cups water

Save the Tomato Juice

Most canned tomatoes are packed in juice or puréed tomato. When you open a can, save juices and add to recipes when liquids are called for. In this recipe, tomato juice from the can could substitute some water used to cook peppers in.

1. Remove tops of red peppers and remove seeds; set aside.

2. Mix kasha and egg white together in small bowl. In large nonstick saucepan sprayed with nonstick cooking spray, add kasha; cook over high heat 2–3 minutes, stirring constantly, until kasha kernels are separated.

3. Add beef broth slowly. Reduce heat; cover and cook 7–10 minutes, until kasha kernels are tender. Transfer to large bowl.

4. Brown beef in small nonstick skillet. Add onions; cook 2–3 minutes, until slightly softened.

5. Add beef mixture and chopped spinach to cooked kasha; mix well. Stir in feta cheese, diced tomato, oregano, and crushed red pepper. Divide mixture equally; stuff each red pepper. Place peppers in 9" × 9" baking dish.

6. Pour water around peppers. Cover with foil; bake in 375°F oven 60–75 minutes, or until peppers are cooked.

Red and White Bean Salad

NUTRITIONAL ANALYSIS (per serving):

Calories: 86   Protein: 8g   Carbohydrates: 27g   Fat: 6g   Saturated Fat: 1g   Cholesterol: 0mg   Sodium: 7mg
Fiber: 7g   PCF Ratio: 17-55-27   Exchange Approx.: 1½ Starches, 1 Vegetable, ½ Very-Lean Meat, 2 Fats

INGREDIENTS | SERVES 8

2 cups navy beans, cooked
2 cups red beans, cooked
1 cup arugula, chopped
¼ cup lemon juice
3 tablespoons olive oil
¼ teaspoon fresh ground pepper
1 cup red onion, thinly sliced
8 ounces cherry tomatoes, cut in half

1. Combine beans together in medium bowl.

2. Whisk together arugula, lemon juice, olive oil, and pepper; pour over beans.

3. Add onions toss lightly to mix. Let mixture refrigerate at least 3 hours.

4. Just before serving, toss in cherry tomatoes; mix lightly.

About Arugula

Arugula has several other names such as rocket, rugula, roquette, and rucola. It is sometimes found in baby greens or mesclun mixes. It has nutty and peppery flavor, which can add interest to a salad or sandwich. Give arugula a try!

Zesty Black Bean Salsa

NUTRITIONAL ANALYSIS (per serving):

Calories: 86   Protein: 3g   Carbohydrates: 12g   Fat: 3g   Saturated Fat: 0g   Cholesterol: 0mg
Sodium: 125mg   Fiber: 4g   PCF Ratio: 15-53-32   Exchange Approx.: ½ Starch, 1 Vegetable, 1 Fat

INGREDIENTS | SERVES 10

1 cup red onion
¼ cup cilantro
¼ cup parsley
1 small jalapeño pepper
1½ cups black beans, cooked
4 cups tomatoes, chopped
3 tablespoons lime juice
2 tablespoons olive oil
Freshly ground black pepper

1. Place onion, cilantro, parsley, and jalapeño in food processor; finely chop.

2. In medium bowl, combine onion mixture, black beans, and tomatoes.

3. In separate small bowl, whisk together lime juice, olive oil, and fresh ground pepper. Pour over beans; mix well. Chill before serving.

Using Canned Beans Versus Cooking Your Own

Canned beans are very convenient and can save you time. Keep in mind sodium content of recipes will be higher with canned beans. Reduce sodium content in canned beans by draining and thoroughly rinsing with cold water before using.

Whole-Wheat Couscous Salad

NUTRITIONAL ANALYSIS (per serving):

Calories: 153 Protein: 4g Carbohydrates: 15g Fat: 9g Saturated Fat: 1g Cholesterol: 0mg
Sodium: 85mg Fiber: 2g PCF Ratio: 9-38-52 Exchange Approx.: 1 Starch, 2 Fats

INGREDIENTS | SERVES 8

1 cup low-sodium chicken broth

¼ cup dried currants

½ teaspoon cumin

¾ cup whole-wheat couscous

¼ cup olive oil

2 tablespoons lemon juice

1 cup broccoli, chopped and steamed to crisp-tender

3 tablespoons pine nuts

1 tablespoon fresh parsley, chopped

1. Combine chicken broth, currants, and cumin; bring to a boil. Remove from heat; stir in couscous. Cover and let sit until cool. Fluff couscous with fork 2–3 times during the cooling process.

2. Whisk together olive oil and lemon juice.

3. Add steamed broccoli and pine nuts to couscous. Pour oil and lemon juice over couscous; toss lightly. Garnish with chopped parsley.

Aren't Currants Just Small Raisins?

Dried currants may look like a miniature raisin, but are actually quite different. Currants are berries from a shrub, not a vine, and there are red and black varieties. Black currants are rich in phytonutrients and antioxidants. They have twice the potassium of bananas and four times the vitamin C of oranges!

CHAPTER 14

Vegetable Sides

Vegetable Broth

NUTRITIONAL ANALYSIS (per serving):

Calories: 10   Protein: 0g   Carbohydrates: 2g   Fat: 0g   Saturated Fat: 0g   Cholesterol: 0mg   Sodium: 8mg
Fiber: 1g   PCF Ratio: 11-85-4   Exchange Approx.: 1 Free Vegetable

INGREDIENTS | YIELDS ABOUT 2½ QUARTS; SERVING SIZE: ¾ CUP

4 carrots, peeled and chopped

2 celery stalks and leaves, chopped

1 green bell pepper, seeded and chopped

2 medium zucchini, chopped

1 small onion, chopped

1 cup chopped fresh spinach

2 cups chopped leeks

½ cup chopped scallions

1 cup chopped green beans

1 cup chopped parsnips

2 bay leaves

2 cloves garlic, crushed

Sea salt and freshly ground black pepper (optional)

3 quarts water

1. Place all of ingredients in large pot; bring to a boil. Reduce heat; cover pan and simmer 30 minutes, or until vegetables are tender. Discard bay leaf.

2. Use slotted spoon to transfer vegetables to different pot; mix with some of broth for Free Exchange vegetable soup. Freeze mixture in single-serving containers to keep on hand for a quick, heat-in-the-microwave snack.

3. Strain remaining vegetables from broth; purée in blender or food processor and return to broth to add dietary fiber and body. Cool and freeze until needed.

Perpetual Broth

The easiest way to create vegetable broth is to keep a container in the freezer for saving liquid from cooked vegetables. Vegetable broth makes a great addition to sauces, soups, and many other recipes. Substitute it for meat broth in most recipes or use instead of water for cooking pasta, rice, and other grains.

Winter Vegetable Casserole

NUTRITIONAL ANALYSIS (per serving):

Calories: 218 Protein: 5g Carbohydrates: 36g Fat: 7g Saturated Fat: 1g Cholesterol: 18mg
Sodium: 392mg Fiber: 5g PCF Ratio: 9-64-27 Exchange Approx.: 1½ Starches, 1½ Vegetables, 1 Fat

INGREDIENTS | SERVES 6

Cooking spray
1½ potatoes, thinly sliced
1½ sweet potatoes, thinly sliced
1 cup parsnips, peeled and sliced
1 cup turnips, sliced
½ cup onions, chopped
3 tablespoons butter
3 tablespoons all-purpose flour
½ teaspoon salt
¼ teaspoon white pepper
1½ cups low-fat milk

1. Spray 2-quart casserole dish with cooking spray.

2. Clean, peel, and slice potatoes, sweet potatoes, parsnips, and turnips; combine. Chop onions and set aside.

3. In small saucepan, melt butter; add flour, salt, and pepper to make a roux. Gradually stir in milk, cooking over low heat; stir well with wire whisk.

4. Bring milk to a boil, stirring constantly, until milk has thickened into a sauce, about 10 minutes. Remove from heat.

5. Arrange ½ of sliced vegetables in casserole dish; top with ½ of chopped onion and white sauce; repeat to make second layer. Cover and cook at 350°F for 45 minutes. Uncover and continue to cook until all vegetables are tender, about 60–70 minutes.

6. Let casserole stand 10 minutes before serving.

Healthy Onion Rings

NUTRITIONAL ANALYSIS (per serving, without salt):

Calories: 111   Protein: 4g   Carbohydrates: 22g   Fat: 1g   Saturated Fat: 0g   Cholesterol: 1mg
Sodium: 255mg   Fiber: 1g   PCF Ratio: 16-80-4   Exchange Approx.: 1 Vegetable, 1 Starch

INGREDIENTS | SERVES 4

1 cup yellow onion slices (¼" thick)
½ cup flour
½ cup nonfat plain yogurt
½ cup bread crumbs
Sea salt and freshly ground black pepper, to taste (optional)

1. Preheat oven to 350°F. Dredge onion slices in flour; shake off any excess. Dip onions in yogurt; dredge through bread crumbs.

2. Prepare baking sheet with nonstick cooking spray. Arrange onion rings on pan; bake 15–20 minutes. Place under broiler for an additional 2 minutes to brown. Season with salt and pepper, if desired.

Oven-Baked Red Potatoes

NUTRITIONAL ANALYSIS (per serving):

Calories: 120   Protein: 2g   Carbohydrates: 26g   Fat: 1g   Saturated Fat: 0g   Cholesterol: 0g
Sodium: 587mg   Fiber: 2g   PCF Ratio: 7-84-9   Exchange Approx.: 1 Starch

INGREDIENTS | SERVES 4

1 pound (16 ounces) small red potatoes, halved

¼ cup fresh lemon juice

1 teaspoon olive oil

1 teaspoon sea salt

¼ teaspoon freshly ground pepper

Preheat oven to 350°F. Arrange potatoes in 13" × 9" ovenproof casserole dish. Combine remaining ingredients; pour over potatoes. Bake 30–40 minutes, or until potatoes are tender, turning 3–4 times to baste.

Remember the Roasting "Rack"

Use caution when roasting potatoes with meat: Potatoes will act like a sponge, soaking up fat. Your best option is to use lean cuts of meat and elevate them and vegetables above fat by putting on a roasting rack in pan or making a "bridge" with celery to elevate meat. Discard celery when done.

Broccoli Raab with Pine Nuts

NUTRITIONAL ANALYSIS (per serving):

Calories: 110   Protein: 5g   Carbohydrates: 6g   Fat: 8g   Saturated Fat: 1g   Cholesterol: 0mg
Sodium: 229mg   Fiber: 4g   PCF Ratio: 18-20-62   Exchange Approx.: 1 Vegetable, 1 Fat

INGREDIENTS | SERVES 4

¾ pound broccoli raab, cooked

1 tablespoon olive oil

4 cloves garlic, chopped

¼ cup sundried tomatoes, chopped

2 tablespoons pine nuts

¼ teaspoon salt

¼ teaspoon crushed red pepper

Preventing Bitter Broccoli Raab

Broccoli raab and other leafy greens (mustard or collard greens) can have a bitter taste once cooked. Rather than add extra salt to offset bitterness, this recipe calls for blanching 2 minutes, which helps reduce bitterness. Blanching should be done as quickly as possible by starting with water at full rolling boil, then removing after 2 minutes of boiling. If allowed to cook too long, boiling process will reduce amount of water-soluble nutrients found in vegetables.

1. Prepare and blanch broccoli before beginning recipe: Rinse well and trim stems. Loosely chop leafy parts, then blanch in 2 quarts boiling water 2 minutes. Drain well.

2. Heat olive oil in large skillet; add garlic. Sauté garlic 1–2 minutes; add cooked broccoli. Toss garlic and broccoli together well, so that oil and garlic are mixed evenly.

3. Add remaining ingredients; cook for an additional 2–3 minutes, until broccoli is tender.

Sweet Potato Crisps

NUTRITIONAL ANALYSIS (per serving, without salt):

Calories: 89 Protein: 1g Carbohydrates: 16g Fat: 2g Saturated Fat: 1g Cholesterol: 0mg
Sodium: 7mg Fiber: 9g PCF Ratio: 6-70-24 Exchange Approx.: 1 Starch, ½ Fat

INGREDIENTS | SERVES 2

1 small sweet potato or yam

1 teaspoon olive oil

Sea salt and freshly ground black pepper, to taste (optional)

1. Preheat oven to 400°F. Scrub sweet potato and pierce flesh several times with fork. Place on microwave-safe plate; microwave 5 minutes on high. Remove from microwave; wrap in aluminum foil. Set aside 5 minutes.

2. Remove foil; peel and cut into French fries. Spread on baking sheet treated with nonstick spray; spritz with olive oil. Bake 10–15 minutes, or until crisp. There's a risk that sweet potato strips will caramelize and burn; check often while cooking to ensure this doesn't occur. Lower oven temperature, if necessary. Season with salt and pepper, if desired.

Sweet Potatoes with Onions and Apple

NUTRITIONAL ANALYSIS:

Calories: 127   Protein: 2g   Carbohydrates: 28g   Fat: 1g   Saturated Fat: 0g   Cholesterol: 1mg
Sodium: 144mg   Fiber: 4g   PCF Ratio: 6-85-9   Exchange Approx.: 1 Starch, ½ Vegetable

INGREDIENTS | SERVES 6

1 pound sweet potatoes (about 2 large)
½ teaspoon canola oil
1 cup onion, thinly sliced
1 apple, peeled and chopped
½ cup low-sodium chicken broth

1. Wash and dry sweet potatoes; pierce skins several times with fork. Microwave on high 5–8 minutes, or until tender.

2. While sweet potatoes are cooling, heat oil in large nonstick skillet over medium-high heat. Add onions; sauté until golden brown, about 10 minutes.

3. Add apple and chicken broth; cook until onions are tender and have caramelized.

4. Scoop cooked sweet potatoes from skins into microwaveable dish; mash lightly. Cover and microwave on high 1–2 minutes, or until potatoes are heated. Top with sautéed onions and serve.

French Tarragon Green Beans

NUTRITIONAL ANALYSIS (per serving, without salt):

Calories: 59   Protein: 0g   Carbohydrates: 5g   Fat: 3g   Saturated Fat: 1g   Cholesterol: 11mg
Sodium: 105mg   Fiber: 1g   PCF Ratio: 3-32-65   Exchange Approx.: 1 Vegetable, 1 Fat

INGREDIENTS | SERVES 4

1½ tablespoons butter
¼ cup red onion, chopped
½ pound fresh green beans
1 tablespoon tarragon, finely chopped

1. Melt butter in nonstick pan. Add onions; sauté until translucent.

2. Add green beans. Cover and steam 2–3 minutes.

3. Add tarragon; combine well. Steam an additional 2–3 minutes.

Oven-Roasted Ratatouille

NUTRITIONAL ANALYSIS (per serving):

Calories: 87　Protein: 2g　Carbohydrates: 11g　Fat: 5g　Saturated Fat: 1g　Cholesterol: 0mg
Sodium: 452mg　Fiber: 3g　PCF Ratio: 9-46-46　Exchange Approx.: 2 Vegetables, 1 Fat

INGREDIENTS | SERVES 12

5 cups eggplant, peeled and cut into ½"
cubes

3 cups yellow squash, cut into ½" pieces

½ pound green beans

½ cup celery, chopped

1 cup red onion, chopped

4 cloves garlic, chopped

1 (28-ounce) can diced tomatoes

1 tablespoon fresh parsley, chopped

¼ teaspoon salt

½ teaspoon rosemary

½ teaspoon thyme

¼ cup olive oil

2 tablespoons balsamic vinegar

1. Preheat oven to 375°F. In large Dutch oven or 9" × 13" baking dish, combine eggplant, yellow squash, green beans, celery, onion, garlic, tomatoes, parsley, salt, rosemary, thyme, and olive oil.

2. Roast uncovered in oven. Stir after 30 minutes, then continue roasting another 30 minutes, or until vegetables are softened and lightly browned on top.

3. Remove from oven. Stir in balsamic vinegar and serve.

Spaghetti Squash and Vegetable Mix

NUTRITIONAL ANALYSIS (per serving):

Calories: 127   Protein: 4g   Carbohydrates: 16g   Fat: 6g   Saturated Fat: 3g   Cholesterol: 5mg
Sodium: 169mg   Fiber: 2g   PCF Ratio: 12-47-41   Exchange Approx.: 1 Starch, 1 Fat

INGREDIENTS | SERVES 6

2 pounds spaghetti squash

Cooking spray

1 cup peas, fresh or frozen

2 tablespoons butter

8 ounces cherry tomatoes, cut in half

1 ounce grated Romano cheese

¼ teaspoon fresh ground pepper

Pasta Alternative

Spaghetti squash is a wonderful alternative to pasta because it is packed with vitamins, minerals, and fiber. While it has a consistency similar to spaghetti, it is much lower in carbohydrates: 1 cup of cooked spaghetti squash has 15g of carbohydrate, while 1 cup of cooked spaghetti has approximately 45g!

1. Cut spaghetti squash in half and scoop out seeds. Spray 9" × 13" baking dish with cooking spray; place squash halves face down. Bake at 400°F for 45 minutes, or until squash is soft-cooked.

2. When squash is cool enough to handle, use a fork to scoop out cooked squash from the outer shell. Scoop into a medium-sized microwaveable bowl.

3. In separate small saucepan, lightly steam peas 2–3 minutes. Add to squash, along with butter; mix well.

4. Place covered bowl in microwave; cook on high 2–3 minutes.

5. Add cherry tomato halves and top with Romano cheese and pepper before serving.

Sesame Snap Peas

NUTRITIONAL ANALYSIS (per serving):

Calories: 49   Protein: 0g   Carbohydrates: 3g   Fat: 4g   Saturated Fat: 0g   Cholesterol: 0mg   Sodium: 149mg
Fiber: 0g   PCF Ratio: 2-27-72   Exchange Approx.: 1 Vegetable, ½ Fat

INGREDIENTS | SERVES 4

½ tablespoon canola oil
10 ounces fresh snap peas
¼ cup scallions, thinly sliced
1 tablespoon fresh grated ginger
2 teaspoons sesame oil
1 tablespoon sesame seeds

1. Heat canola oil in large nonstick skillet or wok.

2. Add snap peas, scallions and ginger; stir-fry until peas are crisp-tender.

3. Stir in sesame oil and sesame seeds; toss lightly and serve.

Amish-Style Turnips

NUTRITIONAL ANALYSIS (per serving):

Calories: 80   Protein: 2g   Carbohydrates: 12g   Fat: 3g   Saturated Fat: 2g   Cholesterol: 40mg
Sodium: 49mg   Fiber: 2g   PCF Ratio: 10-56-34   Exchange Approx.: 1 Vegetable, ½ Starch, ½ Fat

INGREDIENTS | SERVES 6

3 cups turnips, cooked and mashed
½ cup water
1 slice whole-wheat bread
1 tablespoon butter, melted
2 tablespoons Splenda Brown Sugar Blend
½ cup low-fat milk
1 egg

1. Cook turnips in advance. If using fresh turnips, wash, peel, and cut into 1" cubes. Put in covered dish with ½ cup water; microwave on high 10–15 minutes, until tender.

2. Place bread in food processor. Using pulse setting, process until bread is consistency of fine bread crumbs.

3. In medium bowl, mix together bread crumbs, melted butter, Splenda, milk, and egg. Add cooked turnip; mix well.

4. Turn mixture into greased casserole dish. Bake uncovered in 375°F oven for 30–35 minutes.

Greens in Garlic with Pasta

NUTRITIONAL ANALYSIS (per serving, without salt):

Calories: 176   Protein: 8g   Carbohydrates: 26g   Fat: 5g   Saturated Fat: 1g   Cholesterol: 0mg
Sodium: 17mg   Fiber: 3g   PCF Ratio: 17-58-25   Exchange Approx.: 1 Free Vegetable, 1 Fat, 1 Starch, ½ Lean Meat

INGREDIENTS | SERVES 4

2 teaspoons olive oil

4 cloves garlic, crushed

6 cups, tightly packed loose-leaf greens (baby mustard, turnip, chard)

2 cups cooked pasta

2 teaspoons extra-virgin olive oil

¼ cup freshly grated Parmesan cheese

Salt and freshly ground black pepper, to taste (optional)

1. Place sauté pan over medium heat. When hot, add 2 teaspoons of olive oil and garlic. Cook, stirring frequently, until golden brown, 3–5 minutes, being careful not to burn garlic, as that makes it bitter.

2. Add greens; sauté until coated in garlic oil. Remove from heat.

3. In large serving bowl, add pasta, cooked greens, 2 teaspoons of extra-virgin olive oil, and Parmesan cheese; toss to mix. Serve immediately, and season as desired.

Sweet or Salty?

In most cases, when you add a pinch (less than ⅛ teaspoon) of sugar to a recipe, you can reduce the amount of salt without noticing a difference. Sugar acts as a flavor enhancer and magnifies the effect of the salt.

Vegetable Frittata (with Egg Substitute)

NUTRITIONAL ANALYSIS

Calories: 171   Protein: 12g   Carbohydrates: 11g   Fat: 9g   Saturated Fat: 4g   Cholesterol: 195mg
Sodium: 252mg   Fiber: 2g   PCF Ratio: 28-24-48   Exchange Approx.: 1 Vegetable, 1 Lean Meat, 2½ Fats

INGREDIENTS | SERVES 4

1½ tablespoons olive oil

4 ounces red pepper, chopped

3 large eggs

4 ounces egg substitute (or egg whites)

4 ounces asparagus, cut diagonally in 1" pieces

¾ cup potatoes, cooked and cubed

⅓ cup feta cheese, crumbled

1 teaspoon oregano

1. Preheat oven to 350°F. Using ovenproof nonstick skillet, heat olive oil over medium heat. Add red peppers; cook until softened.

2. In medium bowl, beat together eggs and egg substitute. Add asparagus, potatoes, feta, and oregano.

3. Pour eggs into skillet; gently stir until eggs on bottom of pan begin to set. Gently pull cooked eggs from side of skillet, allowing liquid uncooked egg on top to come in contact with heated skillet. Repeat, working all around skillet, until most of eggs on top have begun to set.

4. Transfer skillet to oven; bake until top is set and dry to the touch, about 3–5 minutes. Loosen frittata around edges of skillet and invert onto serving plate.

Crustless Zucchini and Artichoke Quiche

NUTRITIONAL ANALYSIS:

Calories: 224   Protein: 24g   Carbohydrates: 9g   Fat: 10g   Saturated Fat: 4g   Cholesterol: 134mg
Sodium: 798mg   Fiber: 3g   PCF Ratio: 43-16-41   Exchange Approx.: 1 Vegetable, 1½ Lean Meats, 1½ Fats

INGREDIENTS | SERVES 4

Nonstick cooking spray
1 tablespoon olive oil
¼ cup onions, chopped
¾ cup zucchini, grated
1 cup canned artichoke hearts, cut in ½" pieces
1½ cups light Cheddar cheese, grated
2 eggs
½ cup egg whites
½ cup fat-free cottage cheese
¼ teaspoon cayenne
¼ teaspoon salt
⅛ teaspoon fresh-ground pepper

1. Preheat oven to 375°F. Spray 9" pie plate with cooking spray.

2. In large nonstick skillet, heat olive oil; add onion and sauté until translucent.

3. Add zucchini and artichoke hearts; cook additional 3 minutes.

4. Sprinkle grated cheese in bottom of pie plate; add cooked vegetables on top of cheese.

5. In small bowl, whisk eggs, egg whites, cottage cheese, cayenne, salt, and pepper together; pour over vegetables.

CHAPTER 15

Salads

Minted Lentil and Tomato Salad

NUTRITIONAL ANALYSIS

Calories: 136   Protein: 4g   Carbohydrates: 11g   Fat: 9g   Saturated Fat: 1g   Cholesterol: 0mg
Sodium: 211mg   Fiber: 4g   PCF Ratio: 10-31-59   Exchange Approx.: ½ Starch, 1 Vegetable, ½ Lean Meat, 2 Fats

INGREDIENTS | SERVES 6

1 cup dry lentils

2 cups water

½ cup onion, chopped

2 teaspoons garlic, minced

¼ cup celery, chopped

½ cup green pepper, chopped

½ cup parsley, finely chopped

2 tablespoons fresh mint, finely chopped, or 2 teaspoons dried

¼ cup lemon juice

¼ cup olive oil

½ teaspoon salt

1 cup fresh tomato, diced

1. Place lentils and water in medium-sized saucepan; bring to a quick boil. Reduce heat; cover and cook on low 15–20 minutes, or until tender. Drain and transfer to medium bowl.

2. Add onion, garlic, celery, green pepper, parsley and mint; mix well.

3. In small bowl, whisk together lemon juice, olive oil, and salt. Pour into lentils; mix well. Cover and refrigerate several hours.

4. Before serving, mix in diced tomatoes.

Marinated Roasted Peppers and Eggplant

NUTRITIONAL ANALYSIS (per serving):

Calories: 179   Protein: 2g   Carbohydrates: 14g   Fat: 14g   Saturated Fat: 2g   Cholesterol: 0mg
Sodium: 5mg   Fiber: 6g   PCF Ratio: 5-29-66   Exchange Approx.: 3 Vegetables, 3 Fats

INGREDIENTS | SERVES 4

1 pound roasted red peppers

1 large eggplant, sliced into ¼" thick rounds

2 tablespoons olive oil

1 tablespoon balsamic vinegar

2 tablespoons olive oil

1 tablespoon onion, finely chopped

1 teaspoon oregano

Fresh ground pepper

Variations

You can use zucchini or yellow squash in place of eggplant. Other herb choices for the marinade include basil, thyme, or savory. Use marinated vegetables on top of tossed salads or grilled London broil.

1. Follow procedure for roasting red peppers in Chapter 16. Set aside.

2. Brush eggplant slices with 2 tablespoons olive oil; place on grill. Grill on both sides for about 5 minutes each until softened. Remove from grill and place in container. Add roasted peppers to container.

3. Prepare marinade by whisking together balsamic vinegar, 2 tablespoons olive oil, chopped onion, oregano, and pepper; pour over vegetables. Cover and refrigerate.

Spinach Salad with Pomegranate

NUTRITIONAL ANALYSIS (per serving):

Calories: 107   Protein: 4g   Carbohydrates: 8g   Fat: 8g   Saturated Fat: 1g   Cholesterol: 0mg
Sodium: 259mg   Fiber: 3g   PCF Ratio: 13-26-61   Exchange Approx.: 1 Vegetable, 2 Fats

INGREDIENTS | SERVES 6

1 pound fresh spinach
½ cup red onion, very thinly sliced
8 ounces fresh tomatoes, cut into ½"
wedges
⅓ cup walnuts, chopped
½ teaspoon salt
¼ cup lemon juice
1½ tablespoons olive oil
¼ cup pomegranate seeds

1. Wash spinach thoroughly and drain well; loosely chop.

2. Add onions, tomato, and walnuts; toss lightly.

3. In small bowl, whisk together salt, lemon juice, and olive oil. Drizzle over salad; toss lightly.

4. Garnish salad with pomegranate seeds.

For a Different Twist: Toasted Almond Seasoning

Add an extra flavor dimension to salads, rice dishes, or vegetables by sprinkling toasted almonds over the top. Toast ½ cup ground raw almonds in a nonstick skillet over low heat, stirring frequently, until they are a light brown color. Store the cooled almonds in an airtight container in a cool, dry place. This low-sodium substitute has only 16 calories per teaspoon, a PCF Ratio of 14-12-74, and counts as a ½ Fat Exchange Approximation.

Tabbouleh

NUTRITIONAL ANALYSIS (per serving):

Calories: 144   Protein: 3g   Carbohydrates: 15g   Fat: 9g   Saturated Fat: 1g   Cholesterol: 0mg
Sodium: 212mg   Fiber: 4g   PCF Ratio: 7-38-55   Exchange Approx.: ½ Starch, 1 Vegetable, 2 Fats

INGREDIENTS | SERVES 6

1 cup boiling water

½ cup bulgur wheat

1 cup fresh parsley, packed and finely chopped

⅓ cup fresh mint, finely chopped

½ cup red onion, finely chopped

1 cup cucumber, chopped

¼ cup lemon juice

¼ cup olive oil

½ teaspoon salt

Fresh-ground pepper, to taste

1 cup fresh tomato, chopped

2 cups leaf lettuce (optional)

1. In small bowl, pour boiling water over bulgur wheat; let stand 20 minutes.

2. When bulgur is softened, drain and squeeze out any excess water using a colander lined with cheesecloth.

3. Combine parsley, mint, onion, cucumber, and wheat. Add lemon juice, olive oil, salt, and ground pepper; mix well.

4. Cover and refrigerate at least 3 hours.

5. Just before serving, add chopped tomatoes; toss lightly. Serve as is or on bed of leaf lettuce.

Parsley . . . Not Just a Garnish

Parsley is a key ingredient in Tabbouleh and many other Middle Eastern dishes. Parsley is low in calories and packed with Vitamin C, iron, and other trace minerals. Add it liberally to all salads.

Tomato and Cucumber Salad with Mint

NUTRITIONAL ANALYSIS (per serving):

Calories: 68 Protein: 1g Carbohydrates: 7g Fat: 5g Saturated Fat: 1g Cholesterol: 0mg
Sodium: 202mg Fiber: 1g PCF Ratio: 5-32-63 Exchange Approx.: 1 Vegetable, 1 Fat

INGREDIENTS | SERVES 6

2 cucumbers
⅓ cup red wine vinegar
1 teaspoon sugar
½ teaspoon salt
2 cups tomatoes, chopped
⅔ cup red onion, chopped
¼ cup fresh mint, chopped
2 tablespoons olive oil

1. Cut cucumbers in ½" wide pieces; place in medium bowl.

2. Add vinegar, sugar, and salt; stir. Let stand at room temperature for 15 minutes.

3. Add tomatoes, red onion, mint, and olive oil; toss lightly to blend.

Tomatoes Stuffed with Quinoa Salad

NUTRITIONAL ANALYSIS (per serving):

Calories: 180   Protein: 5g   Carbohydrates: 24g   Fat: 9g   Saturated Fat: 2g   Cholesterol: 4mg
Sodium: 78mg   Fiber: 4g   PCF Ratio: 11-49-40   Exchange Approx.: ½ Starch, 2½ Vegetables, 2½ Fats

INGREDIENTS | SERVES 6

½ cup quinoa

1 cup water

6 large (3 pounds) tomatoes

1½ cups cucumber, peeled and finely diced

⅓ cup fresh parsley, chopped

¼ cup fresh mint, chopped

½ cup red onion, finely chopped

3 tablespoons feta cheese, crumbled

2 tablespoons lemon juice

3 tablespoons olive oil

1. Rinse quinoa in fine mesh strainer before cooking. To cook: place quinoa and water in small saucepan; bring to a boil. Reduce heat; cover and cook until all water is absorbed, about 15 minutes. Cool.

2. Prepare tomatoes: remove caps and hollow out, leaving shell about ½" thick.

3. In mixing bowl, combine quinoa, cucumbers, parsley, mint, red onion, and feta cheese.

4. Mix lemon juice and olive oil together; pour over quinoa and vegetables.

5. Stuff tomatoes with mixture and serve.

Cucumbers with Minted Yogurt

NUTRITIONAL ANALYSIS (per serving):

Calories: 31   Protein: 2g   Carbohydrates: 4g   Fat: 1g   Saturated Fat: 0g   Cholesterol: 2mg
Sodium: 52mg   Fiber: 1g   PCF Ratio: 27-56-17   Exchange Approx.: 1 Vegetable

INGREDIENTS | SERVES 8

1 cup nonfat plain yogurt

1 clove garlic, finely chopped

¼ teaspoon cumin

1 teaspoon lemon zest

½ cup mint

1 tablespoon lemon juice

¼ teaspoon salt

4 cups cucumbers, seeded and chopped

1. Combine yogurt, garlic, cumin, lemon zest, mint, lemon juice, and salt in blender or food processor; blend until smooth.

2. Add yogurt mixture to cucumbers; mix. Chill before serving.

Wilted Lettuce with a Healthier Difference

NUTRITIONAL ANALYSIS (per serving):

Calories: 71   Protein: 2g   Carbohydrates: 7g   Fat: 5g   Saturated Fat: 1g   Cholesterol: 0mg
Sodium: 9mg   Fiber: 2g   PCF Ratio: 8-34-57   Exchange Approx.: 2 Free Vegetables, 1 Fat

INGREDIENTS | SERVES 1

½ teaspoon olive oil

¼ cup chopped red onion

1½ cups tightly packed loose-leaf lettuce

¼ teaspoon lemon juice or your choice of vinegar

½ teaspoon extra-virgin olive oil, walnut oil, or almond oil

Optional seasonings to taste:

Dried herbs of your choice, such as thyme or parsley

Pinch of sugar

Pinch of toasted sesame seeds or grated Parmesan cheese

1. In heated nonstick skillet treated with nonstick spray, add ½ teaspoon of olive oil and all red onion. Sauté until onion is almost transparent; add greens. Sauté greens until warmed and wilted.

2. In salad bowl, whisk lemon juice with ½ teaspoon oil. Add pinch of herbs and sugar, if using; whisk into oil mixture. Add wilted greens; toss with dressing. Top salad with pinch of toasted sesame seeds or Parmesan cheese, if desired. Serve immediately.

Adventuresome Additions

Dried cranberries or other dried fruit are delicious in wilted lettuce dishes; the addition of diced apples or pineapple makes a perfect wilted greens accompaniment for pork.

Mandarin Snap Pea Salad

NUTRITIONAL ANALYSIS (per serving, without dressing):

Calories: 76   Protein: 4g   Carbohydrates: 16g   Fat: 0g   Saturated Fat: 0g   Cholesterol: 0mg
Sodium: 344mg   Fiber: 4g   PCF Ratio: 19-78-3   Exchange Approx.: ½ Starch, 1 Vegetable, ½ Lean Meat, ½ Fat

INGREDIENTS | SERVES 8

¾ pound snap peas, cut into ½" pieces

1 cup canned mandarin oranges, drained

1½ cups canned kidney beans, rinsed and drained

1 cup red onion, thinly sliced

½ cup fresh parsley, chopped

2 cups cabbage, chopped

⅓ cup poppy seed dressing (recipe below)

1. In medium bowl, combine snap peas, mandarin oranges, kidney beans, onions, parsley, and cabbage.

2. Mix in poppy seed dressing; refrigerate several hours before serving.

Poppy Seed Dressing

Combine ½ cup red wine vinegar, ¼ cup orange juice, 3 tablespoons lemon juice, ½ cup canola oil, 1 teaspoon Splenda brown sugar blend, 1 teaspoon dry mustard, 1 teaspoon salt, and 1 tablespoon poppy seeds; mix well in covered jar. Store in refrigerator. Nutritional Analysis 1 ounce serving (1½ tablespoons): 68 Calories; Protein: 0g; Carbohydrates: 9g; Fat: 7g; Saturated Fat: 1g; Cholesterol: 0mg; Sodium: 148mg; PCF Ration: 1-9-90; Exchange Approx.: 1½ Fats

Broccoli-Cauliflower Slaw

NUTRITIONAL ANALYSIS (per serving):

Calories: 117   Protein: 6g   Carbohydrates: 13g   Fat: 5g   Saturated Fat: 1g   Cholesterol: 0mg
Sodium: 46mg   Fiber: 1g   PCF Ratio: 19-42-39   Exchange Approx.: 1 Misc. Carbohydrate, 1 Fat

INGREDIENTS | SERVES 8

4 cups raw broccoli flowerets

4 cups raw cauliflower

½ cup real mayonnaise

1 cup cottage cheese, 1% fat

3 tablespoons tarragon vinegar

1 tablespoon balsamic vinegar

⅛ cup packed brown sugar

3 tablespoons red onion

1. Put broccoli and cauliflower in food processor; pulse-process to consistency of shredded cabbage. Pour into a bowl.

2. Place remaining ingredients in food processor; process until smooth. Pour resulting dressing over broccoli-cauliflower mixture; stir. Chill until ready to serve.

Tip

Substituting cottage cheese for some mayonnaise cuts fat and calories considerably. Cut them even more by using nonfat cottage cheese and mayonnaise.

Zesty Feta and Olive Salad

NUTRITIONAL ANALYSIS (per serving):

Calories: 109   Protein: 3g   Carbohydrates: 6g   Fat: 8g   Saturated Fat: 3g   Cholesterol: 132mg
Sodium: 326mg   Fiber: 2g   PCF Ratio: 11-22-66   Exchange Approx.: 1 Vegetable, 2 Fats

INGREDIENTS | SERVES 4

2 ounces crumbled feta

1 small red onion, diced

½ cup chopped celery

½ cup diced cucumber

1 clove garlic, minced

1 teaspoon lemon zest

1 teaspoon orange zest

1 cup halved very small cherry tomatoes

½ cup mix of green and kalamata olives, pitted and sliced

1 tablespoon extra-virgin olive oil

2 tablespoons minced fresh Italian parsley

2 teaspoons minced fresh oregano

1 teaspoon minced fresh mint

1 tablespoon minced fresh cilantro (optional)

Large romaine or butter lettuce leaves

Freshly ground black pepper

1. In a large bowl, place feta, onion, celery, cucumber, garlic, lemon zest, orange zest, tomatoes, and olives; mix.

2. Add olive oil and fresh herbs; toss again.

3. Arrange lettuce leaves on 4 salad plates; spoon feta salad on top. Top with pepper and serve.

Avocado and Peach Salad

NUTRITIONAL ANALYSIS (per serving, without salt):

Calories: 160   Protein: 2g   Carbohydrates: 15g   Fat: 11g   Saturated Fat: 2g   Cholesterol: 0mg
Sodium: 11mg   Fiber: 4g   PCF Ratio: 6-35-59   Exchange Approx.: 3 Fats, 1 Free Vegetable, ½ Fruit

---

INGREDIENTS | SERVES 4

⅛ cup water

⅛ cup frozen orange juice concentrate

1 clove garlic, crushed

1 teaspoon rice wine vinegar

1 tablespoon extra-virgin olive oil

½ teaspoon vanilla

1½ cups tightly packed baby arugula

2 tablespoons tarragon leaves

1 avocado, peeled and diced

1 peach, peeled and diced

½ cup thinly sliced Vidalia onion

Kosher or sea salt and freshly ground black pepper, to taste (optional)

1. In measuring cup, whisk water, orange juice concentrate, garlic, vinegar, oil, and vanilla together until well mixed.

2. Prepare salad by arranging layers of arugula and tarragon, then avocado, peach, and onions, then drizzle with prepared orange juice vinaigrette. Season with salt and pepper, if desired, and serve.

Experiment Sensibly

When it comes to new herbs and spices, err on the side of caution. Not sure whether or not you like a seasoning: mix all other ingredients together and test a bite of salad with pinch of herb or spice before adding it to entire recipe.

Orange-Avocado Slaw

NUTRITIONAL ANALYSIS (per serving, without salt):

Calories: 60   Protein: 2g   Carbohydrates: 5g   Fat: 5g   Saturated Fat: 1g   Cholesterol: 0mg
Sodium: 14mg   Fiber: 2g   PCF Ratio: 11-27-62   Exchange Approx.: 1 Fat, ½ Free Vegetable

INGREDIENTS | SERVES 10

¼ cup orange juice

½ teaspoon curry powder

⅛ teaspoon ground cumin

¼ teaspoon sugar

1 teaspoon white wine vinegar

1 tablespoon olive oil

1 avocado, peeled and chopped

5 cups broccoli slaw mix

Sea salt and freshly ground black pepper, to taste (optional)

1. In bowl, whisk together orange juice, curry powder, cumin, sugar, and vinegar. Add oil in stream, whisking until emulsified.

2. In large bowl, toss avocado with slaw mix; drizzle with vinaigrette. Chill until ready to serve. Season with salt and pepper, if desired.

Spinach Salad with Apple-Avocado Dressing

NUTRITIONAL ANALYSIS (per serving):

Calories: 122   Protein: 2g   Carbohydrates: 8g   Fat: 10g   Saturated Fat: 1g   Cholesterol: 0mg
Sodium: 90mg   Fiber: 3g   PCF Ratio: 7-25-68   Exchange Approx.: 2½ Fats, 1 Free Vegetable

INGREDIENTS | SERVES 4

¼ cup unsweetened apple juice

1 teaspoon (or up to 1 tablespoon) cider vinegar

1 clove garlic, minced

1 teaspoon Bragg's Liquid Aminos or soy sauce

½ teaspoon Worcestershire sauce (see recipe for homemade in Chapter 16)

2 teaspoons olive oil

1 avocado, peeled and chopped

2½ cups tightly packed spinach and other salad greens

½ cup thinly sliced red onion

½ cup sliced radishes

½ cup bean sprouts

1. In blender or food processor, combine juice, vinegar (the amount of which will depend on how you like your dressing), garlic, Liquid Aminos, Worcestershire, oil, and avocado; process until smooth.

2. In large bowl, toss greens, onions, radishes, and bean sprouts. Pour dressing over salad; toss again.

Salads Don't Have to Be Fat Free

Unless on a calorie-restricted diet, fat free may not be the best choice—consult your dietitian. Vegetable oils—combined with a diet rich in fish, fruits, vegetables, whole grains, and nuts—are much healthier than using chemically created fat-free foods and are believed to prevent certain cancers, too.

Taco Salad

NUTRITIONAL ANALYSIS (per serving):

Calories: 426   Protein: 23g   Carbohydrates: 58g   Fat: 13g   Saturated Fat: 7g   Cholesterol: 30mg   Sodium: 380mg
Fiber: 13g   PCF Ratio: 21-53-26   Exchange Approx.: 1 Lean Meat, 1 High-Fat Meat, 3 Starches, 2 Vegetables

INGREDIENTS | SERVES 8

1 recipe Turkey Chili (see Chapter 10)

8 cups tightly packed salad greens

8 ounces Cheddar cheese, shredded (to yield 2 cups)

8 ounces nonfat corn chips

Nonstarchy free-exchange vegetables of your choice, such as chopped celery, onion, or banana or jalapeño peppers (optional)

1. Prepare Turkey Chili.

2. Divide salad greens between 8 large bowls. Top with chili, Cheddar cheese, corn chips, and vegetables or peppers, if using.

Rainbow Potato Salad

NUTRITIONAL ANALYSIS (per serving):

Calories: 146   Protein: 5g   Carbohydrates: 29g   Fat: 2g   Saturated Fat: 0g   Cholesterol: 0mg
Sodium: 615mg   Fiber: 5g   PCF Ratio: 12-77-11   Exchange Approx.: 1½ Starches

INGREDIENTS | SERVES 6

2 pounds red potatoes (6 medium)

⅓ cup carrots, finely chopped

¼ cup onion, finely chopped

¼ cup green pepper, finely chopped

¼ cup yellow or red bell pepper, finely chopped

2 tablespoons red wine vinegar

2 tablespoons lemon juice

¼ teaspoon celery seed

1 teaspoon sugar

½ teaspoon salt

2 tablespoons light mayonnaise

1. Wash and scrub red potatoes. Place whole potatoes in pot and cover with water. Boil over medium heat for about 20 minutes until potatoes are cooked. Drain; set aside to cool.

2. Combine carrots, onion, peppers, vinegar, lemon juice, celery seed, sugar, and salt in small bowl; mix. Cover and refrigerate for 2–3 hours.

3. After vegetables have marinated, add light mayonnaise; mix well.

4. Cut potatoes (with skins on) into ½" cubes.

5. In large bowl, combine potatoes and vegetables; mix well.

Potato and Snow Pea Salad

NUTRITIONAL ANALYSIS (per serving):

Calories: 139   Protein: 5g   Carbohydrates: 28g   Fat: 1g   Saturated Fat: 0g   Cholesterol: 3mg
Sodium: 223mg   Fiber: 3g   PCF Ratio: 13-78-9   Exchange Approx.: 1 Starch, 1 Vegetable, ½ Fat

INGREDIENTS | SERVES 8

2 pounds red potatoes (6 medium)
3 slices bacon
½ cup onion, chopped
¾ pound snow peas, cut in ½" pieces
½ teaspoon salt
¼ cup apple cider vinegar

1. Wash and scrub red potatoes. Place whole potatoes in pot; cover with water. Boil over medium heat for 20 minutes until potatoes are cooked. Drain and chill. Once chilled, cut into ½" cubes.

2. Cut bacon slices into ½" pieces. Place in nonstick fry pan with onions; fry for 3-4 minutes until crisp. There should be a light coating of fat in pan from bacon. If there is excess fat, pour off before going to step 3.

3. Add snow peas; toss with bacon and onion mixture for 2 minutes. Remove from heat.

4. Dissolve salt into cider vinegar; mix into snow peas.

5. In large bowl, combine potatoes and snow peas; mix well.

Summer Salad

NUTRITIONAL ANALYSIS (per serving):

Calories: 73   Protein: 2g   Carbohydrates: 7g   Fat: 5g   Saturated Fat: 1g   Cholesterol: 0mg
Sodium: 109mg   Fiber: 2g   PCF Ratio: 9-36-55   Exchange Approx.: 1 ½ Vegetables, 1 Fat

INGREDIENTS | SERVES 6

2 cups snap peas, cut into 1" pieces

2 cups summer squash, cut into ½" pieces

½ cup carrots, chopped

3 tablespoons mushrooms, minced

2 cups cucumbers, chopped

¼ cup onion, thinly sliced

2 tablespoons canola oil

2 tablespoons balsamic vinegar

¼ teaspoon salt

¼ teaspoon thyme

¼ teaspoon marjoram

1. Combine snap peas, squash, carrots and mushrooms; steam for 2–3 minutes, until crisp-tender. Cool and refrigerate.

2. When cooled, add cucumbers and onions.

3. Whisk together canola oil, balsamic vinegar, salt, thyme, and marjoram. Pour over vegetables; toss lightly. Serve.

Tip

Add the oil and vinegar dressing just before serving. Minimize the exposure of vinegar to certain vegetables such as snap peas or green beans to retain their bright colors.

CHAPTER 16

Salad Dressings, Salsas, and Sauces

Creamy Feta Vinaigrette

NUTRITIONAL ANALYSIS

Calories: 31   Protein: 1g   Carbohydrates: 1g   Fat: 2g   Saturated Fat: 1g   Cholesterol: 4mg
Sodium: 57mg   Fiber: 0g   PCF Ratio: 17-17-66   Exchange Approx.: ½ Fat

INGREDIENTS | YIELDS ABOUT ⅔ CUP; SERVING SIZE: 1 TABLESPOON

½ cup plain low-fat yogurt

1 tablespoon lemon juice

1 tablespoon olive oil

1½ ounces feta cheese

2 teaspoons mint

½ packet Splenda (optional)

Fresh-ground pepper, to taste

Process all ingredients in food processor or blender. Chill before serving.

Raspberry Tarragon Vinaigrette

NUTRITIONAL ANALYSIS (per serving):

Calories: 120   Protein: 0g   Carbohydrates: 9g   Fat: 9g   Saturated Fat: 1g   Cholesterol: 0mg
Sodium: 0mg   Fiber: 0g   PCF Ratio: 0-33-67   Exchange Approx.: 2 Fats

INGREDIENTS | YIELDS ¾ CUP; SERVING SIZE: 1 TABLESPOON

½ cup olive oil

¼ cup raspberry vinegar (see recipe below)

2 teaspoons lemon juice

½ tablespoon tarragon, finely chopped

Salt and pepper, to taste

Combine ingredients in a covered jar; shake thoroughly.

Making Raspberry Vinegar

Combine 2 cups raspberries, lightly mashed; 2 tablespoons honey; and 2 cups red wine vinegar in nonstick saucepan. Simmer uncovered for 10 minutes; cool. Place in 1-quart jar; store at room temperature for 3 weeks. Strain vinegar from berries; pour strained vinegar into an empty wine bottle. Cork or cap.

Bleu Cheese Dressing

NUTRITIONAL ANALYSIS (per serving):

Calories: 24   Protein: 1g   Carbohydrates: 1g   Fat: 2g   Saturated Fat: 1g   Cholesterol: 3mg
Sodium: 52mg   Fiber: 0g   PCF Ratio: 21-23-57   Exchange Approx.: ½ Fat

INGREDIENTS | YIELDS 6 TABLESPOONS; SERVING SIZE: 1 TABLESPOON

2 tablespoons plain nonfat yogurt

1 tablespoon cottage cheese

1 tablespoon real mayonnaise

½ teaspoon lemon juice

½ teaspoon honey

1 tablespoon plus 2 teaspoons crumbled bleu cheese

Put yogurt, cottage cheese, mayonnaise, lemon juice, and honey in blender; process until smooth. Fold in bleu cheese.

Dijon Vinaigrette

NUTRITIONAL ANALYSIS (per serving):

Calories: 74   Protein: 0g   Carbohydrates: 1g   Fat: 8g   Saturated Fat: 1g   Cholesterol: 0mg
Sodium: 266mg   Fiber: 0g   PCF Ratio: 1-2-97   Exchange Approx.: 2 Fats

INGREDIENTS | YIELDS ABOUT 5 TABLESPOONS; SERVING SIZE: 1 TABLESPOON

1 tablespoon Dijon mustard
½ teaspoon sea salt
½ teaspoon freshly ground black pepper
1 tablespoon red wine vinegar
3 tablespoons virgin olive oil

Put all ingredients in small bowl; use wire whisk or fork to mix.

The Vinegar–Oil Balancing Act

The easiest way to tame too much vinegar is to add some vegetable oil. Because oil adds fat, the better alternative is to start with less vinegar and add it gradually until you arrive at a flavor you prefer.

Tangy Lemon-Garlic Tomato Dressing

NUTRITIONAL ANALYSIS (per serving):

Calories: 7   Protein: 0g   Carbohydrates: 1g   Fat: 1g   Saturated Fat: 0g   Cholesterol: 0mg
Sodium: 1mg   Fiber: 1g   PCF Ratio: 14-44-42   Exchange Approx.: ½ Free

INGREDIENTS | YIELDS ABOUT ¾ CUP; SERVING SIZE: 1 TABLESPOON

1 tablespoon ground flaxseeds
2 cloves garlic
⅛ cup cider vinegar
⅛ teaspoon freshly ground pepper
1 small tomato, chopped
¼ teaspoon celery seed
1 tablespoon lemon juice
¼ cup water

Place all ingredients in blender; blend until smooth.

Friendly Fat and Fiber

In addition to providing fiber, ground flax-seeds are rich sources of omega-3 and -6 essential fatty acids. The oil is low in saturated fat and therefore a heart-healthy choice. Just remember that flaxseed oil must be refrigerated or it will go rancid.

Lemon-Almond Dressing

NUTRITIONAL ANALYSIS (per serving):

Calories: 25   Protein: 1g   Carbohydrates: 2g   Fat: 2g   Saturated Fat: 0g   Cholesterol: 0mg
Sodium: 0mg   Fiber: 1g   PCF Ratio: 12-27-61   Exchange Approx.: ½ Fat

INGREDIENTS | YIELDS ABOUT ⅔ CUP; SERVING SIZE: 1 TABLESPOON

¼ cup raw almonds

1 tablespoon lemon juice

¼ cup water

1½ teaspoons honey

¼ teaspoon lemon pepper

½ slice (1" diameter) peeled ginger

¼ clove garlic

1½ teaspoons chopped fresh chives, or ½ teaspoon dried chives

1½ teaspoons chopped fresh sweet basil, or ½ teaspoon dried basil

Put all ingredients in food processor or blender; process until smooth.

Salad: Undressed

Make a quick salad without dressing by mixing chopped celery, onion, and other vegetables such as cucumbers or zucchini. Add low-salt seasoning or toss vegetables with Bragg's Liquid Aminos or low-sodium soy sauce and serve over salad greens.

Caribbean Kiwi Salsa

NUTRITIONAL ANALYSIS

Calories: 79   Protein: 2g   Carbohydrates: 19g   Fat: 0g   Saturated Fat: 0g   Cholesterol: 0mg
Sodium: 28mg   Fiber: 3g   PCF Ratio: 9-87-5   Exchange Approx.: 1 Fruit, ½ Vegetable

INGREDIENTS | SERVES 6

1 cup kiwi, peeled and chopped
1 cup pineapple, chopped
1 cup mango, peeled and chopped
⅓ cup red onion, chopped
1 cup red bell pepper, chopped
⅓ cup black beans, cooked
3 tablespoons fresh cilantro, chopped
2 tablespoons lime juice
½ teaspoon chili powder
Dash cayenne

1. Mix all ingredients together in medium bowl.

2. Chill at least 2 hours before serving.

Zesty Black Bean Salsa

NUTRITIONAL ANALYSIS (per serving, without salt):

Calories: 91   Protein: 4g   Carbohydrates: 13g   Fat: 3g   Saturated Fat: 0g   Cholesterol: 0mg
Sodium: 125mg   Fiber: 4g   PCF Ratio: 15-55-30   Exchange Approx.: ½ Starch, 1 Vegetable, ½ fat

INGREDIENTS | SERVES 10

1 cup red onion, chopped
¼ cup cilantro, chopped
¼ cup parsley, chopped
3 tablespoons jalapeño, chopped
1½ cups black beans, cooked
4 cups tomato, chopped
3 tablespoons lime juice
2 tablespoons olive oil

1. Place onion, cilantro, parsley, and jalapeño in food processor; chop finely.

2. In medium bowl, combine onion mixture, black beans, and tomatoes.

3. In small bowl, whisk together lime juice and olive oil. Pour over ingredients; mix well.

4. Chill well before serving.

Fresh Peach-Mango Salsa

NUTRITIONAL ANALYSIS (per serving):

Calories: 45   Protein: 1g   Carbohydrates: 10g   Fat: 1g   Saturated Fat: 0g   Cholesterol: 0mg
Sodium: 104mg   Fiber: 2g   PCF Ratio: 9-82-9   Exchange Approx.: ½ Fruit

INGREDIENTS | SERVES 6

1 cup mango, peeled and cut into ¼"
pieces

1 peach, peeled and cut into ¼" pieces

1 cup red onion, finely chopped

1 cup cucumber, peeled and cut into ¼"
pieces

1 tablespoon balsamic vinegar

1 tablespoon lime juice

1 teaspoon chili powder

½ teaspoon cumin

1 tablespoon fresh cilantro, chopped

1 tablespoon parsley, chopped

¼ teaspoon salt

1. Mix all ingredients together in medium bowl.

2. Chill at least 4 hours before serving.

Roasted Corn Salsa

NUTRITIONAL ANALYSIS

Calories: 104   Protein: 4g   Carbohydrates: 24g   Fat: 1g   Saturated Fat: 0g   Cholesterol: 0mg
Sodium: 77mg   Fiber: 3g   PCF Ratio: 12-80-8   Exchange Approx.: 1 Starch, ½ Vegetable

INGREDIENTS | SERVES 6

2 ears corn

1½ cups fresh tomatoes, skinned and chopped

½ cup red onion, chopped

3 tablespoons jalapeño pepper, finely chopped

1 tablespoon rice wine vinegar

¼ cup roasted red pepper, chopped

1½ tablespoons cilantro, chopped

1 teaspoon garlic, finely chopped

1 tablespoon lime juice

½ teaspoon cumin

2 teaspoons red wine vinegar

1. Husk corn and place on grill. Cook for about 10-12 minutes until lightly browned and tender. Set aside to cool.

2. Combine tomatoes, onion, jalapeño, rice wine vinegar, red pepper, cilantro, garlic, lime juice, cumin, and vinegar.

3. When corn has cooled, cut kernels off cob and add to remaining ingredients.

Cranberry Orange Relish

NUTRITIONAL ANALYSIS (per serving):

Calories: 62   Protein: 0g   Carbohydrates: 16g   Fat: 0g   Saturated Fat: 0g   Cholesterol: 0mg
Sodium: 3mg   Fiber: 2g   PCF Ratio: 3-96-1   Exchange Approx.: 1 Fruit

INGREDIENTS | SERVES 12; SERVING SIZE ½ CUP

16 ounces fresh cranberries

1½ cups orange sections

2 teaspoons orange zest

¼ cup brown sugar

⅓ cup Splenda Granular

1 teaspoon cinnamon

1. Chop cranberries and orange sections in food processor using pulse setting until coarsely chopped. Transfer to saucepan.

2. Bring cranberry mixture, orange zest, brown sugar, and Splenda to boil over medium heat. Cook for 2 minutes.

3. Remove from heat, stir in cinnamon. Chill before serving.

Horseradish Mustard

NUTRITIONAL ANALYSIS (per serving):

Calories: 10   Protein: 0g   Carbohydrates: 1g   Fat: 1g   Saturated Fat: 0g   Cholesterol: 0mg
Sodium: 68mg   Fiber: 0g   PCF Ratio: 12-25-63   Exchange Approx.: 1 Free Condiment

INGREDIENTS | YIELDS ¾ CUP; SERVING SIZE: 1 TEASPOON

¼ cup dry mustard

2½ tablespoons prepared horseradish

1 teaspoon sea salt

¼ cup white wine vinegar

1 tablespoon olive oil

Cayenne pepper, to taste (optional)

Combine ingredients in food processor or blender; process until smooth. Pour into decorative jar; store in refrigerator.

Roasting Red Peppers

The traditional method of roasting a red pepper is to use a long-handled fork to hold the pepper over the open flame of a gas burner until it is charred. Of course, there are a variety of other methods as well. You can place the pepper on a rack set over an electric burner and turn it occasionally, until the skin is blackened. This should take about 4 to 6 minutes. You can also put the pepper over direct heat on a preheated grill. Use tongs to turn the pepper occasionally. Another method is to broil the pepper on a broiler rack about 2 inches from the heat, turning the pepper every 5 minutes. Total broiling time will be about 15 to 20 minutes, or until the skins are blistered and charred. The key to peeling the peppers is letting them sit in their steam in a closed container until they are cool. Once the peppers are cool, the skin will rub or peel off easily.

Cranberry-Raisin Chutney

NUTRITIONAL ANALYSIS (per serving, without salt):

Calories: 14   Protein: 0g   Carbohydrates: 3g   Fat: 0g   Saturated Fat: 0g   Cholesterol: 0mg
Sodium: 1mg   Fiber: 0g   PCF Ratio: 4-93-3   Exchange Approx.: 1 Free Condiment

INGREDIENTS | **YIELDS ABOUT 3 CUPS;
SERVING SIZE:
1 TABLESPOON**

1 cup diced onions

1 cup diced peeled apples

1 cup diced bananas

1 cup diced peaches

¼ cup raisins

¼ cup dry white wine

¼ cup dried cranberries

¼ cup apple cider vinegar

1 teaspoon brown sugar

Sea salt and freshly ground black pepper, to taste (optional)

In large saucepan, combine all ingredients. Cook over low heat for about 1 hour, stirring occasionally. Cool completely. Can be kept for a week in refrigerator or in freezer for 3 months, or canned using same sterilizing method you'd use to can mincemeat.

Tip

This chutney is also good if you substitute other dried fruit for the raisins or cranberries, such as using the dried Fancy Fruit Mix from Nutty Guys (*www.nuttyguys.com*).

Roasted Red Pepper and Plum Sauce

NUTRITIONAL ANALYSIS (per serving):

Calories: 38   Protein: 0g   Carbohydrates: 10g   Fat: 1g   Saturated Fat: 0g   Cholesterol: 0mg
Sodium: 76mg   Fiber: 1g   PCF Ratio: 3-95-2   Exchange Approx.: ½ Misc. Carbohydrate

INGREDIENTS | YIELDS 2 CUPS; SERVING SIZE: 1 TABLESPOON

1 large roasted red pepper, pulp only (see sidebar)

½ pound apricots, quartered and pitted

¾ pound plums, quartered and pitted

1⅓ cups apple cider vinegar

⅔ cup water

⅓ cup white sugar

½ cup brown sugar

2 tablespoons corn syrup

2 tablespoons fresh grated ginger

1 teaspoon salt

1 tablespoon toasted mustard seeds

4 scallions, chopped (white part only)

1 teaspoon minced garlic

½ teaspoon ground cinnamon

1. Place all ingredients together in large pot; bring to a boil. Reduce heat; simmer, covered, for 30 minutes.

2. Uncover and simmer for another hour.

3. Place in blender or food processor; process to desired consistency. Can be stored in refrigerator for 4–6 weeks.

Roasting Red Peppers

The traditional method of roasting a red pepper is to use a long-handled fork to hold the pepper over the open flame of a gas burner until it is charred. Of course, there are a variety of other methods as well. You can place the pepper on a rack set over an electric burner and turn it occasionally, until the skin is blackened. This should take about 4 to 6 minutes. You can also put the pepper over direct heat on a preheated grill. Use tongs to turn the pepper occasionally. Another method is to broil the pepper on a broiler rack about 2 inches from the heat, turning the pepper every 5 minutes. Total broiling time will be about 15 to 20 minutes, or until the skins are blistered and charred. The key to peeling the peppers is letting them sit in their steam in a closed container until they are cool. Once the peppers are cool, the skin will rub or peel off easily.

Homemade Worcestershire Sauce

NUTRITIONAL ANALYSIS (per serving):

Calories: 14   Protein: 0g   Carbohydrates: 4g   Fat: 0g   Saturated Fat: 0g   Cholesterol: 0mg
Sodium: 15mg   Fiber: 0g   PCF Ratio: 3-97-0   Exchange Approx.: 1 Free Condiment

INGREDIENTS | YIELDS 1 CUP; SERVING SIZE: 1 TABLESPOON

1½ cups cider vinegar

¼ cup plum jam

1 tablespoon blackstrap molasses

1 clove garlic, crushed

⅛ teaspoon chili powder

⅛ teaspoon ground cloves

Pinch of cayenne pepper

¼ cup chopped onion

½ teaspoon ground allspice

⅛ teaspoon dry mustard

1 teaspoon Bragg's Liquid Aminos

Combine all ingredients in large saucepan; stir until mixture boils. Lower heat; simmer uncovered for 1 hour, stirring occasionally. Store in covered jar in refrigerator.

Pesto Sauce

NUTRITIONAL ANALYSIS (per serving):

Calories: 37   Protein: 1g   Carbohydrates: 1g   Fat: 4g   Saturated Fat: 1g   Cholesterol: 1mg
Sodium: 14mg   Fiber: 0g   PCF Ratio: 10-6-85   Exchange Approx.: 1 Fat

---

INGREDIENTS | YIELDS ABOUT 3 CUPS; SERVING SIZE: 1 TABLESPOON

¾ cup pine nuts
4 cups tightly packed basil leaves
½ cup freshly grated Parmesan cheese
3 large garlic cloves, minced
¼ teaspoon salt
1 teaspoon freshly ground black pepper
½ cup extra-virgin olive oil

1. Preheat oven to 350°F. Spread pine nuts on baking sheet. Bake for about 5 minutes; stir. Continue to bake for 10 minutes until nuts are golden brown and highly aromatic, stirring occasionally. Let nuts cool completely; chop finely.

2. Fill medium-sized heavy saucepan halfway with water. Place over medium heat; bring to a boil. Next to pot, place large bowl filled with water and ice. Using tongs, dip a few basil leaves into boiling water. Blanch for 3 seconds; quickly remove from boiling water and place in ice water. Repeat process until all basil has been blanched, adding ice to water as needed. Drain basil in colander and pat dry with a towel.

3. In blender or food processor, combine basil, pine nuts, cheese, garlic, salt, pepper, and all but 1 tablespoon olive oil; process until smooth and uniform. Pour into airtight container and add remaining olive oil to top to act as protective barrier. Pesto can be stored in refrigerator for up to 5 days.

4. To freeze pesto, place it in a tightly sealed container. To freeze small amounts of pesto, pour into ice cube trays and freeze until solid. Once frozen, you can remove the pesto cubes and place them in sealed freezer bags.

Mock Cream

NUTRITIONAL ANALYSIS (per recipe):

Calories: 147   Protein: 14g   Carbohydrates: 21g   Fat: 1g   Saturated Fat: 1g   Cholesterol: 8mg
Sodium: 221mg   Fiber: 0g   PCF Ratio: 39-57-3   Exchange Approx.: 1½ Skim Milks

INGREDIENTS | YIELDS 1¼ CUPS;
SERVING SIZE:
2 TABLESPOONS

1 cup skim milk
¼ cup nonfat dry milk

Process ingredients in blender until mixed. Use as a substitute for heavy cream.

Comparative Analysis

Using 1¼ cups heavy cream would give you the following breakdown: Calories: 515.02; Protein: 3.06g; Carbohydrates: 4.17g; Fat: 55.27g; Saturated Fat: 34.40g; Cholesterol: 204.79mg; Sodium: 56.16mg; Fiber: 0.00g; PCF Ratio: 2-3-95; Exchange Approx.: 11 Fats.

Mock White Sauce

NUTRITIONAL ANALYSIS (per recipe):

Calories: 61   Protein: 2g   Carbohydrates: 6g   Fat: 3g   Saturated Fat: 2g   Cholesterol: 9mg
Sodium: 190mg   Fiber: 0g   PCF Ratio: 20-36-44   Exchange Approx.: ½ Fat, ½ Skim Milk

INGREDIENTS | YIELDS ABOUT 1 CUP; SERVING SIZE: ½ CUP

1 tablespoon unsalted butter
1 tablespoon flour
¼ teaspoon sea salt
Pinch of white pepper
1 cup Mock Cream (Chapter 16)

1. In medium-sized heavy nonstick saucepan, melt butter over very low heat. Butter should gently melt; you do not want it to bubble and turn brown. While butter is melting, mix together flour, salt, and white pepper in small bowl.

2. Once butter is melted, add flour mixture; stir constantly. (A heat-safe flat-bottom spoon safe for nonstick pans works well for this.) Once mixture thickens and starts to bubble, about 2 minutes, slowly pour in some Mock Cream; stir until blended with roux. Add a little more Mock Cream; stir until blended. Add remaining Mock Cream; continue cooking, stirring constantly to make sure sauce doesn't stick to bottom of pan. Once sauce begins to steam and appears it's just about to boil, reduce heat and simmer until sauce thickens, or about 3 minutes.

Fat-Free Roux

NUTRITIONAL ANALYSIS (per serving, Roux only):

Calories: 13 Protein: 0g Carbohydrates: 2g Fat: 0g Saturated Fat: 0g Cholesterol: 0mg
Sodium: 1mg Fiber: 0g PCF Ratio: 1-99-0 Exchange Approx.: 1 Free

INGREDIENTS | YIELDS ENOUGH TO THICKEN 1 CUP OF LIQUID; SERVING SIZE: ¼ CUP

1 tablespoon cornstarch
2 tablespoons wine
Make this roux with red wine for a defatted beef broth gravy. Use white wine for chicken or seafood gravy or sauce.

1. Whisk ingredients together until well blended, making sure there are no lumps.

2. To use as thickener for 1 cup of broth, heat broth until it reaches a boil. Slowly whisk cornstarch-wine mixture into broth; return to a boil. Reduce heat; simmer, stirring constantly, until mixture thickens enough to coat back of spoon. (A gravy or sauce made in this manner will thicken more as it cools. It's important to bring a cornstarch slurry to a boil; this helps it thicken and removes the starchy taste.)

CHAPTER 17

Salt-Free Spice Mixes

Herbal and Other Seasoning Blends

Using herbs is a delicious way to season dishes and cut the amount of salt needed for flavor, too. Although fresh herbs need to be used immediately, dried herb mixtures can be prepared in advance and stored in an airtight container.

The easiest way to dry fresh herbs is to put the baking sheet in an oven at 200 to 225°F for 1 hour. Blends made from whole seeds or leaves usually need to be coarsely ground in a spice grinder or small food processor prior to using.

Try mixing up a few different spice blends to have on hand. Making your own blends saves time and money. Herbs and spices have no significant caloric value, and since they are made without salt, there is no sodium.

Barbecue Blend

- 4 tablespoons dried basil
- 4 tablespoons dried rubbed sage
- 4 tablespoons dried thyme
- 4 teaspoons cracked black pepper
- 4 teaspoons dried savory
- 1 teaspoon dried lemon peel

Cajun Blend

- 2 tablespoons paprika
- 1½ tablespoons garlic powder
- 1 tablespoon onion powder
- ½ tablespoon black pepper
- 2 teaspoons cayenne pepper
- 2 teaspoons dried oregano
- 2 teaspoons dried thyme

Caribbean Blend

- 1 tablespoon curry powder
- 1 tablespoon ground cumin
- 1 tablespoon ground allspice
- 1 tablespoon ground ginger
- 1 teaspoon ground cayenne pepper

Country Blend

- 5 teaspoons dried thyme
- 4 teaspoons dried basil
- 4 teaspoons dried chervil
- 4 teaspoons dried tarragon

Fish and Seafood Blend

- 5 teaspoons dried basil
- 5 teaspoons crushed fennel seed
- 4 teaspoons dried parsley
- 1 teaspoon dried lemon peel

French Blend

- 1 tablespoon crushed dried tarragon
- 1 tablespoon crushed dried chervil
- 1 tablespoon onion powder

Herbes de Provence Blend

- 4 teaspoons dried oregano
- 2 teaspoons dried basil
- 2 teaspoons dried sweet marjoram
- 2 teaspoons dried thyme

- 1 teaspoon dried mint
- 1 teaspoon dried rosemary
- 1 teaspoon dried sage leaves
- 1 teaspoon fennel seed
- 1 teaspoon dried lavender (optional)

Italian Blend

- 1 tablespoon crushed dried basil
- 1 tablespoon crushed dried thyme
- 1 tablespoon crushed dried oregano
- 2 tablespoons garlic powder

Mediterranean Blend

- 1 tablespoon dried sun-dried tomatoes
- 1 tablespoon dried basil
- 1 teaspoon dried oregano
- 1 teaspoon dried thyme
- 1 tablespoon garlic powder

Middle Eastern Blend

- 1 tablespoon ground coriander
- 1 tablespoon ground cumin
- 1 tablespoon turmeric
- 1 teaspoon ground cinnamon
- 1 teaspoon crushed dried mint

Old Bay Seasoning

- 1 tablespoon celery seed
- 1 tablespoon whole black peppercorns
- 6 bay leaves
- ½ teaspoon whole cardamom
- ½ teaspoon mustard seed
- 4 whole cloves
- 1 teaspoon sweet Hungarian paprika
- ¼ teaspoon mace

Pacific Rim Blend

- 1 tablespoon Chinese five-spice powder
- 1 tablespoon paprika
- 1 tablespoon ground ginger
- 1 teaspoon black pepper

Sonoran Blend

- 1 tablespoon ground chili powder
- 1 tablespoon black pepper
- 1 tablespoon crushed dried oregano
- 1 tablespoon crushed dried thyme
- 1 tablespoon crushed dried coriander
- 1 tablespoon garlic powder

Stuffing Blend

- 6 tablespoons dried rubbed sage
- 3 tablespoons dried sweet marjoram
- 2 tablespoons dried parsley
- 4 teaspoons dried celery flakes

Texas Seasoning Blend

- 3 tablespoons dried cilantro
- 2 tablespoons dried oregano
- 4 teaspoons dried thyme
- 2 tablespoons pure good-quality chili powder
- 2 tablespoons freshly ground black pepper
- 2 tablespoons ground cumin
- 2 small crushed dried chili peppers
- 1 teaspoon garlic powder

CHAPTER 18

Breads and Muffins

Basic White Bread

NUTRITIONAL ANALYSIS (per serving):

Calories: 77   Protein: 2g   Carbohydrates: 15g   Fat: 1g   Saturated Fat: 0g   Cholesterol: 0mg
Sodium: 175mg   Fiber: 1g   PCF Ratio: 11-79-10   Exchange Approx.: 1 Starch

INGREDIENTS | YIELDS 2 LARGE LOAVES; SERVING SIZE: 1 SLICE

5½–6 cups flour

1 package (2½ teaspoons) active dry yeast

¼ cup warm water

2 tablespoons sugar

1¾ cups warm potato water or plain water

2 tablespoons shortening

1 tablespoon sea salt

1. Place ⅓ of flour in large bowl and set aside. Mix yeast with ¼ cup warm water in another bowl, stirring well. Add sugar and potato water to yeast. Add mixture to flour; stir well. Set aside 5 minutes to allow yeast to proof.

2. Stir; cut in shortening using a pastry blender or your hands. Stir in salt and as much of remaining flour as possible. Dough has enough flour when it's still somewhat sticky to the touch, yet pulls away from side of bowl as it's stirred. Turn dough onto lightly floured work surface. Knead for 8–10 minutes, until smooth and elastic, adding flour as necessary. Dough will take on an almost glossy appearance once it's been kneaded sufficiently.

3. Transfer dough to bowl treated with nonstick spray. Cover with damp cloth; place in warm, draft-free area. Allow to rise until double in volume, about 1–1½ hours.

4. Punch dough down and let rise a second time, until almost doubled in bulk.

5. Treat two 9" × 5" bread pans with nonstick spray. Punch dough down again; divide into 2 loaves. Shape loaves; place in bread pans. Cover and let rise until almost doubled.

6. Preheat oven to 350°F. Bake 20–30 minutes, or until golden brown. Remove from pans and allow to cool on rack.

Fiber-Enriched Cheddar Bread

NUTRITIONAL ANALYSIS (per serving):

Calories: 141   Protein: 6g   Carbohydrates: 25g   Fat: 1g   Saturated Fat: 0g   Cholesterol: 2mg
Sodium: 546mg   Fiber: 1g   PCF Ratio: 19-73-8   Exchange Approx.: 1½ Starches

INGREDIENTS | YIELDS 1 LOAF (12 SLICES); SERVING SIZE: 1 SLICE

1½ cups warm water

1 package (2½ teaspoons) active dry yeast

2½ teaspoons salt

½ cup wheat bran

3 cups bread flour

⅔ cups reduced-fat Cheddar cheese, grated

1 tablespoon Parmesan cheese

Cornmeal for cookie sheet

1. Combine water, yeast, and salt in mixer bowl or food processor. Add remaining ingredients; mix well using dough hook or dough attachment until very soft dough is formed.

2. Transfer dough to large, loosely covered bowl; allow to rise at room temperature for 2 hours. Dough can be used after rising, but is much easier to handle after it has been refrigerated several hours or overnight.

3. When ready to bake, sprinkle a light dusting of flour on top of dough. With floured hands, remove dough from bowl; shape into round loaf.

4. Place dough on cookie sheet or pizza peel liberally covered with cornmeal. Allow dough to rise at room temperature for 45 minutes.

5. Preheat oven to 450°F with baking or pizza stone placed in center rack of oven. Before transferring dough to hot stone, slash dough across top using floured sharp knife. Slide dough onto hot baking stone; place shallow pan of hot water on lower rack of oven to create steam underneath bread.

6. Bake for 40 minutes, or until bread is deeply browned and has a hardened crust. Remove to a cooling rack; allow to cool before slicing.

Golden Raisin Bread

NUTRITIONAL ANALYSIS (per serving):

Calories: 163   Protein: 6g   Carbohydrates: 34g   Fat: 1g   Saturated Fat: 0g   Cholesterol: 0mg
Sodium: 497mg   Fiber: 3g   PCF Ratio: 13-82-5   Exchange Approx.: 1½ Starches; ½ Fruit

INGREDIENTS | YIELDS 1 LOAF (12 SLICES); SERVING SIZE: 1 SLICE

1½ cups warm water

2½ teaspoons active dry yeast

2½ teaspoons salt

⅓ cup wheat germ

1 cup whole-wheat flour

2 cups bread flour

2 tablespoons honey

1 teaspoon cinnamon

½ cup golden raisins

1 tablespoon egg white

½ tablespoon water

Tools of the Trade

Nonstick pans with dark surface absorb too much heat, which causes breads to burn. Chicago Metallic makes muffin, mini-muffin, and other bread pans with lighter-colored Silverstone nonstick coating that are much better suited for baking.

1. Combine water, yeast, and salt in mixer bowl or food processor. Using dough hook or dough attachment for food processor, add in remaining ingredients except egg white and water; mix well until very soft dough is formed.

2. Transfer dough to loosely covered large bowl; allow to rise at room temperature for 2 hours. Dough can be used after rising; however, it is much easier to handle after it has been refrigerated several hours or overnight.

3. When ready to bake, lightly grease 9" × 4" × 3" loaf pan. Scoop dough out of bowl with wet hands (this makes it easier to handle); shape into elongated loaf and place in loaf pan. Allow dough to rise for 1 hour.

4. Preheat oven to 375°F. Brush loaf with egg wash of 1 tablespoon of egg white and ½ tablespoon water.

5. Bake on middle rack of preheated oven. Place shallow pan of hot water on the lower rack to create steam under bread.

6. Bake for 45–50 minutes, until bread is golden brown. Cool in pan for 10 minutes, then remove to wire rack. Allow bread to cool completely before slicing.

Whole-Wheat Bread

NUTRITIONAL ANALYSIS (per serving):

Calories: 86   Protein: 2g   Carbohydrates: 17g   Fat: 1g   Saturated Fat: 0g   Cholesterol: 0mg
Sodium: 118mg   Fiber: 1g   PCF Ratio: 10-77-13   Exchange Approx.: 1 Starch

**INGREDIENTS | YIELDS 2 LOAVES;
SERVING SIZE: 1 SLICE**

1 package (2½ teaspoons) active
dry yeast

2 cups warm water

3 cups unbleached all-purpose or bread
flour

2 tablespoons sugar

½ cup hot water

2 teaspoons salt

½ cup brown sugar

3 tablespoons shortening

3 cups whole-wheat flour

History Lesson

The sponge process of making bread was
more popular years ago, when foodstuffs
were less processed and the quality of
yeast was less reliable. The yeast works in a
batter and the dough rises only once. The
sponge process produces a loaf that is
lighter but coarser grained.

1. Add yeast to 2 cups warm water. Stir in all-purpose
   flour and sugar; beat until smooth, either by hand or
   with mixer. Set in warm place to proof until it
   becomes foamy and bubbly, up to 1 hour.

2. Combine ½ cup hot water, salt, brown sugar, and
   shortening; stir. Allow to cool to lukewarm. (Stirring
   sugar until it's dissolved should be sufficient to cool
   water; test to be sure, as adding liquid that's too warm
   can kill yeast.) Add to bubbly flour mixture. Stir in
   whole-wheat flour; beat until smooth, but do not
   knead.

3. Divide dough into 2 lightly greased pans. Cover; set in
   warm place until doubled in size. Preheat oven to
   350°F; bake for 50 minutes.

Honey Oat Bran Bread

NUTRITIONAL ANALYSIS (per serving):

Calories: 86   Protein: 3g   Carbohydrates: 16g   Fat: 1g   Saturated Fat: 0g   Cholesterol: 8mg
Sodium: 109mg   Fiber: 1g   PCF Ratio: 15-72-13   Exchange Approx.: 1 Starch

INGREDIENTS | YIELDS 1 LARGE LOAF; SERVING SIZE: 1 SLICE

1¼ cups skim milk

2 tablespoons nonfat buttermilk powder

1 tablespoon olive or canola oil

1 medium egg

1 cup oat bran

1 teaspoon sea salt

½ cup whole-wheat flour

2½ cups unbleached all-purpose or bread flour

1 tablespoon honey

1 package (2½ teaspoons) active dry yeast

Use light-crust setting on your bread machine; add ingredients in order recommended by manufacturer. Be careful yeast doesn't come in contact with salt.

7-Grain Bread

NUTRITIONAL ANALYSIS (per serving):

Calories: 82   Protein: 3g   Carbohydrates: 15g   Fat: 1g   Saturated Fat: 0g   Cholesterol: 8mg
Sodium: 108mg   Fiber: 1g   PCF Ratio: 14-73-12   Exchange Approx.: 1 Starch

**INGREDIENTS | YIELD: 1 LARGE LOAF;
SERVING SIZE: 1 SLICE**

1¼ cups skim milk

2 tablespoons nonfat milk powder

1 tablespoon olive or canola oil

¾ cup dry 7-grain cereal

½ cup oat bran

1 teaspoon sea salt

2¼ cups unbleached all-purpose or
bread flour

½ cup whole-wheat flour

1 tablespoon honey

1 package (2½ teaspoons) dry yeast

Add ingredients to bread machine in order recommended by manufacturer; careful that yeast doesn't come in contact with salt. Bake on whole-wheat bread setting.

Lactose-Free Bread

When cooking for someone who is lactose intolerant, substitute equal amounts of water or soy milk for any milk called for in bread recipes.

Multigrain Cornbread

NUTRITIONAL ANALYSIS (per serving):

Calories: 124   Protein: 4g   Carbohydrates: 20g   Fat: 3g   Saturated Fat: 1g   Cholesterol: 16mg
Sodium: 220mg   Fiber: 2g   PCF Ratio: 12-65-23   Exchange Approx.: 1 Starch, ½ Fat

INGREDIENTS | SERVES 16; SERVING SIZE: 1 SLICE

Nonstick cooking spray
1 egg
2 tablespoons egg whites
3 tablespoons butter, melted
1½ cups low-fat buttermilk
1 teaspoon vanilla
1¾ cups cornmeal
¾ cup whole-wheat pastry flour
1 tablespoon ground flax seed
3 tablespoons Splenda Granulated
1 tablespoon sugar
4 teaspoons baking powder
½ teaspoon baking soda
Pinch salt

1. Preheat oven to 375°F. Spray 8" × 8" square baking pan with nonstick cooking spray.

2. In medium bowl, whisk together egg, egg whites, butter, buttermilk, and vanilla. Set aside.

3. In larger bowl, combine cornmeal, flour, flax seed, Splenda, sugar, baking powder, baking soda, and salt; mix well.

4. Make well in center of dry ingredients; pour in buttermilk mixture. Mix gently with spoon until all dry ingredients are moistened; do not over mix.

5. Spoon batter into prepared pan. Bake for 25–30 minutes, or until center springs back when lightly touched. Cool on wire rack before slicing into pieces.

Don't Have Buttermilk?

Soured milk is a good substitution for buttermilk in baking. To replace 1 cup of buttermilk in a recipe, stir 1 tablespoon of white vinegar or fresh lemon juice into 1 cup of milk. Let the milk stand for 5 minutes, or until milk thickens.

Cheddar Cornbread

NUTRITIONAL ANALYSIS (per serving):

Calories: 102   Protein: 3g   Carbohydrates: 16g   Fat: 3g   Saturated Fat: 2g   Cholesterol: 8mg
Sodium: 172mg   Fiber: 1g   PCF Ratio: 13-63-24   Exchange Approx.: 1 Starch, ½ Fat

INGREDIENTS | YIELDS 1 LARGE LOAF;
SERVING SIZE: 1 SLICE

1¼ cups water

1 tablespoon honey

3 tablespoons butter

¼ cup nonfat milk powder

1 package (2½ teaspoons) active
dry yeast

2½ cups unbleached all-purpose or
bread flour

1 cup yellow cornmeal

1½ teaspoons sea salt

⅔ cup grated Cheddar cheese

1. Use light-crust setting. Add all ingredients except cheese in order suggested by bread machine manual. Process on basic bread cycle according to manufacturer's directions.

2. At beeper (or end of first kneading), add cheese.

Cottage Cheese Bread

NUTRITIONAL ANALYSIS (per serving):

Calories: 76 Protein: 3g Carbohydrates: 13g Fat: 1g Saturated Fat: 1g Cholesterol: 11mg
Sodium: 114mg Fiber: 1g PCF Ratio: 16-68-16 Exchange Approx.: 1 Starch

INGREDIENTS | YIELDS 1 LARGE LOAF;
SERVING SIZE: 1 SLICE

¼ cup water

1 cup nonfat cottage cheese

2 tablespoons butter

1 egg

1 tablespoon sugar

¼ teaspoon baking soda

1 teaspoon salt

3 cups unbleached all-purpose or bread flour

1 package (2½ teaspoons) active dry yeast

Add ingredients in order recommended by manufacturer, being careful yeast doesn't come in contact with salt. Check bread machine at "beep" to make sure dough is pulling away from sides of pan and forming a ball. Add water or flour, if needed. (Note: You do not want dough to be overly dry.) Bake at white bread setting, light crust.

Why Breads Need Salt

Salt is only used in bread to enhance the flavor. If salt comes directly in contact with yeast before yeast has had a chance to begin to work, it can hinder the action of the yeast. Keep that in mind when adding ingredients to your bread machine.

Hawaiian-Style Bread

NUTRITIONAL ANALYSIS (per serving):

Calories: 89   Protein: 2g   Carbohydrates: 17g   Fat: 1g   Saturated Fat: 1g   Cholesterol: 11mg
Sodium: 103mg   Fiber: 1g   PCF Ratio: 11-75-14   Exchange Approx.: 1 Starch

INGREDIENTS | YIELDS 1 LARGE LOAF, 24 SLICES; SERVING SIZE: 1 SLICE

1 egg

½ cup pineapple juice, or ⅛ cup frozen pineapple juice concentrate and ⅜ cup water

¾ cup water

2 tablespoons butter

1 teaspoon vanilla

½ teaspoon dried ginger

1 teaspoon salt

1½ cups unbleached bread flour

2⅛ cups unbleached all-purpose flour

¼ cup sugar

2 tablespoons nonfat milk powder

1 package (2½ teaspoons) active dry yeast

Unless instructions for bread machine differ, add ingredients in order listed here. Use light-crust setting.

Fiber-Enriched Banana Bread

NUTRITIONAL ANALYSIS (per serving):

Calories: 65   Protein: 5g   Carbohydrates: 29g   Fat: 4g   Saturated Fat: 1g   Cholesterol: 22mg
Sodium: 348mg   Fiber: 4g   PCF Ratio: 12-67-21   Exchange Approx.: 1 Starch, ½ Fruit, 1 Fat

INGREDIENTS | YIELDS 1 LARGE LOAF, 12 SLICES; SERVING SIZE: 1 SLICE

Nonstick cooking spray
½ cup buttermilk
¼ cup wheat bran
1 cup mashed ripe banana
1 egg
¼ cup egg whites
2 tablespoons canola oil
1 teaspoon vanilla
2 tablespoons honey
1¼ cups whole-wheat pastry flour
½ cup all-purpose flour
⅓ cup Splenda Granulated
1 teaspoon baking soda
1½ teaspoons baking powder
½ teaspoon salt

1. Preheat oven to 375°F. Spray 9" × 4" × 3" loaf pan with nonstick cooking spray.

2. Place buttermilk and wheat bran in medium bowl; allow wheat bran to soak 10 minutes. Stir in banana, egg, egg whites, oil, vanilla, and honey.

3. In larger bowl, sift together flours, Splenda, baking soda, baking powder, and salt; add dry ingredients to banana mixture. Using a large spoon, stir just until dry ingredients are moistened; do not over mix.

4. Spoon batter into prepared loaf pan. Bake for 45 minutes, or until top is lightly browned and inserted toothpick comes out clean. Cool in pan for 10 minutes before removing to wire rack.

Whole-Wheat Zucchini Bread

NUTRITIONAL ANALYSIS (per serving):

Calories: 178   Protein: 4g   Carbohydrates: 29g   Fat: 6g   Saturated Fat: 1g   Cholesterol: 25mg
Sodium: 243mg   Fiber: 3g   PCF Ratio: 9-63-28   Exchange Approx.: 1½ Starches, 1 Fat

INGREDIENTS | YIELDS 4 MINI LOAVES, 20 SLICES (5 SLICES PER MINI LOAF); SERVING SIZE: 1 SLICE

Cooking spray
2 eggs
2 tablespoons egg whites
½ cup honey
2 cups zucchini, shredded
⅔ cup unsweetened applesauce
⅓ cup canola oil
2 teaspoons vanilla
2 cups whole-wheat pastry flour
1 cup all-purpose flour
¼ cup Splenda Granulated
1 teaspoon salt
2 teaspoons baking powder
1 teaspoon baking soda
2 teaspoons cinnamon
½ teaspoons nutmeg
⅓ cup sunflower seeds, toasted

1. Preheat oven to 350°F. Spray 4 aluminum mini loaf pans with cooking spray.

2. In large mixing bowl, beat egg and egg whites until foamy. Mix in honey, zucchini, applesauce, canola oil, and vanilla.

3. In separate mixing bowl, sift together whole-wheat flour, all-purpose flour, Splenda, salt, baking powder, baking soda, cinnamon, and nutmeg.

4. Gradually add dry ingredients to zucchini mixture; mix until all ingredients are combined, but do not over mix. Stir in sunflower seeds.

5. Divide batter evenly into prepared mini loaf pans. Bake for 35–40 minutes, or until tops are browned and inserted toothpick comes out clean.

6. Remove pans to wire rack and cool for 10 minutes before removing from pans. Cool completely before slicing.

Variations

For variation to this recipe, ⅓ cup dried cranberries, currants, raisins, or chopped nuts can be added in place of the sunflower seeds.

Applesauce Buckwheat Muffins

NUTRITIONAL ANALYSIS (per muffin, with crisp topping):

Calories: 182   Protein: 5g   Carbohydrates: 27g   Fat: 7g   Saturated Fat: 1g   Cholesterol: 24mg
Sodium: 302mg   Fiber: 3g   PCF Ratio: 11-56-34   Exchange Approx.: 1 Starch, ½ Fruit, 1 Fat

**INGREDIENTS | YIELDS 12 MUFFINS;
SERVING SIZE: 1 MUFFIN**

1 cup buttermilk

½ cup applesauce, unsweetened

¼ cup canola oil

1 egg

2 tablespoons egg whites

2 tablespoons maple syrup

1 teaspoon vanilla

1¼ cups whole-wheat pastry flour

¾ cup light buckwheat flour

¼ cup Splenda granular

1½ teaspoons baking powder

1½ teaspoons baking soda

¼ teaspoon salt

2 teaspoons cinnamon

¼ teaspoon allspice

Crisp Topping (optional):

1 tablespoon Splenda Brown Sugar
Blend

¼ teaspoon cinnamon

¼ cup oats

2 teaspoons ground flax seed

1 tablespoon whole-wheat pastry flour

1 tablespoon butter, melted

1. Preheat oven to 375°F. Prepare muffin pan with nonstick cooking spray.

2. In medium bowl, whisk together buttermilk, applesauce, oil, egg, egg whites, maple syrup, and vanilla.

3. In separate bowl, sift together whole-wheat flour, buckwheat flour, Splenda, baking powder, baking soda, salt, and spices. Gradually add dry ingredients to liquid mixture; mix just enough to combine ingredients. Do not over mix. Spoon batter evenly into prepared muffin pan.

4. In small bowl, mix together all ingredients for crisp topping. Sprinkle evenly on top of each muffin.

5. Bake for 20–25 minutes, or until center of muffin springs back when lightly touched. Cool in muffin tin for 5 minutes before removing to wire rack.

Pear Walnut Muffins

NUTRITIONAL ANALYSIS (per muffin, with crisp topping):

Calories: 195   Protein: 5g   Carbohydrates: 27g   Fat: 8g   Saturated Fat: 1g   Cholesterol: 24mg   Sodium: 289mg   Fiber: 3g   PCF Ratio: 11-54-35   Exchange Approx.: 1 Starch, ½ Fruit, 1 Fat

INGREDIENTS | 12 MUFFINS; SERVING SIZE: 1 MUFFIN

1 cup buttermilk

3 tablespoons canola oil

1 egg

2 tablespoons egg whites

⅔ cup pears, peeled and chopped

2 tablespoons honey

1¼ cups whole-wheat pastry flour

¾ cup all-purpose flour

3 tablespoons Splenda Granulated

1½ teaspoons baking powder

1½ teaspoons baking soda

¼ teaspoon salt

1 teaspoon cinnamon

¼ teaspoon ginger

⅓ cup walnuts, chopped

Crisp Topping (optional):

1 tablespoon Splenda Brown Sugar Blend

Pinch ginger

¼ cup oats

2 teaspoons ground flax seed

1 tablespoon whole-wheat pastry flour

1 tablespoon butter, melted

1. Preheat oven to 375°F. Prepare muffin pan with nonstick cooking spray.

2. In medium bowl. whisk together buttermilk, oil, egg, egg whites, pears, and honey.

3. In separate bowl, sift together whole-wheat flour, all-purpose flour, Splenda, baking powder, baking soda, salt, spices, and walnuts. Gradually add dry ingredients to liquid mixture; stir just enough to combine ingredients. Do not over mix. Spoon batter evenly into prepared muffin pan.

4. In small bowl, mix together all ingredients for crisp topping. Sprinkle evenly on top of each muffin.

5. Bake for 20–25 minutes, or until center of muffin springs back when lightly touched. Cool in muffin tin for 5 minutes before removing to wire rack.

Whole-Wheat Pastry Flour

Whole-wheat pastry flour is a finer grind of soft white wheat. When used in quick bread and muffin recipes, it delivers more nutrition and fiber than white flour and yields a lighter texture than whole-wheat flour.

Angelic Buttermilk Batter Biscuits

NUTRITIONAL ANALYSIS (per serving):

Calories: 74   Protein: 2g   Carbohydrates: 12g   Fat: 2g   Saturated Fat: 1g   Cholesterol: 6mg
Sodium: 55mg   Fiber: 1g   PCF Ratio: 11-64-26   Exchange Approx.: 1 Starch

INGREDIENTS | YIELDS 24 BISCUITS; SERVING SIZE: 1 BISCUIT

3 tablespoons nonfat buttermilk powder
2 tablespoons granulated sugar
¾ cup warm water
1 tablespoon active dry yeast
2½ cups unbleached all-purpose flour
½ teaspoon sea salt
½ teaspoon baking powder
¼ cup unsalted butter
¼ cup nonfat plain yogurt

Why Breads Need Sugar

Bread recipes need sugar or sweetener, like honey, to "feed" the yeast. This helps the yeast work, which in turn helps the bread rise.

1. Put buttermilk powder, sugar, and warm water in food processor; process until mixed. Sprinkle yeast over top; pulse once or twice to mix. Allow mixture to sit at room temperature for about 5 minutes, or until yeast begins to bubble. Add all remaining ingredients to food processor; pulse until mixed, being careful not to over process the dough.

2. Preheat oven to 400°F; drop 1 heaping teaspoon per biscuit onto baking sheet treated with nonstick spray. Set tray in warm place; allow biscuits to rise for about 15 minutes.

3. Bake biscuits for 12–15 minutes.

Orange Date Bread

NUTRITIONAL ANALYSIS (per serving):

Calories: 79   Protein: 2g   Carbohydrates: 16g   Fat: 1g   Saturated Fat: 0g   Cholesterol: 8mg
Sodium: 130mg   Fiber: 1g   PCF Ratio: 9-80-10   Exchange Approx.: 1 Starch

INGREDIENTS | YIELDS 2 LARGE LOAVES; SERVING SIZE: 1 SLICE

2 tablespoons frozen orange juice concentrate

2 tablespoons orange zest

¾ cup pitted, chopped dates

½ cup brown sugar

¼ cup granulated sugar

1 cup plain nonfat yogurt

1 egg

1¼ cups all-purpose flour

¾ cup whole-wheat flour

1 teaspoon baking soda

1 teaspoon baking powder

½ teaspoon salt

1 tablespoon vegetable oil

1 teaspoon vanilla extract

1. Preheat oven to 350°F. Spray 4 mini-loaf pans with nonfat cooking spray.

2. In food processor, process orange juice concentrate, orange zest, dates, sugars, yogurt, and egg until mixed. (This will cut dates into smaller pieces, too.) Add remaining ingredients; pulse until mixed, scraping down side of bowl if necessary.

3. Divide mixture between the pans. Spread the mixture so each pan has an even layer. Bake for 15–20 minutes, or until a toothpick inserted into center of loaf comes out clean.

4. Cool bread in pans on wire rack for 10 minutes. Remove bread to rack and cool to room temperature.

Are Your Eyes Bigger Than Your Stomach?

Use mini–loaf pans. It's much easier to arrive at the number of servings in the form of a full slice when you use smaller loaf pans. There's a psychological advantage to getting a full rather than half slice.

CHAPTER 19

Reduced-Carbohydrate Desserts

Glazed Carrot Cake

NUTRITIONAL ANALYSIS (per serving):

Calories: 149   Protein: 5g   Carbohydrates: 28g   Fat: 2g   Saturated Fat: 1g   Cholesterol: 42mg
Sodium: 220mg   Fiber: 2g   PCF Ratio: 13-74-13   Exchange Approx.: 1 Starch, ½ Vegetable, 1 Fruit

INGREDIENTS | SERVES 9

1½ cups unbleached all-purpose flour

1 teaspoon baking powder

1 teaspoon baking soda

1½ teaspoons cinnamon

¼ teaspoon ground cloves

¼ teaspoon ground allspice

⅛ teaspoon ground nutmeg

1 tablespoon sugar

⅛ cup (2 tablespoons) frozen, unsweetened apple juice concentrate

2 eggs

¼ cup water

2 tablespoons ground flaxseed

1 teaspoon vanilla

3 tablespoons nonfat plain yogurt

1 cup canned unsweetened crushed pineapple, ¼ cup of liquid retained

1 cup finely shredded carrots

¼ cup seedless raisins

Glaze

⅛ cup (2 tablespoons) frozen, unsweetened apple juice concentrate

1 tablespoon water

1. Preheat oven to 350°F. Sift together dry ingredients and spices.

2. Using food processor or mixer, blend sugar, apple juice concentrate, and eggs until well mixed. Stir water and flaxseed together in small microwave-safe bowl; microwave on high for 30 seconds, then stir. (Mixture should be consistency of egg whites; if it isn't, microwave at 15-second increments until it is.) Gradually beat into egg mixture, along with vanilla, yogurt, and ¼ cup pineapple liquid.

3. Stir in dry ingredients. Fold in pineapple (drained of any remaining juice), carrots, and raisins.

4. Treat 8" baking pan with nonstick spray. Spoon mixture into pan; bake for 20–25 minutes. Allow cake to cool slightly while you prepare glaze.

5. Mix apple juice concentrate and water until concentrate is melted. (You can microwave the mixture for 15–20 seconds, if necessary.) Spread evenly over cake.

Mock Whipped Cream

NUTRITIONAL ANALYSIS (per serving):

Calories: 24   Protein: 1g   Carbohydrates: 2g   Fat: 1g   Saturated Fat: 0g   Cholesterol: 1mg
Sodium: 17mg   Fiber: 0g   PCF Ratio: 21-41-38   Exchange Approx.: ½ Fat

---

**INGREDIENTS | YIELDS 3½ CUPS;
SERVING SIZE:
2 TABLESPOONS**

1 envelope Knox Unflavored Gelatine

¼ cup cold water

½ cup hot water

2 tablespoons almond oil

3 tablespoons powdered sugar

1 teaspoon vanilla

1 cup ice water

1¼ cups nonfat milk powder

Know Your Ingredients

"Gelatine" is the name of the commercial Knox Unflavoured Gelatine product used to make gelatin. Although any unflavored gelatin will work, the nutritional analyses for all recipes are based on the Knox brand.

1. Allow gelatin to soften in cold water; pour into blender. Add hot water; blend for 2 minutes, until gelatin is dissolved.

2. While continuing to blend mixture, gradually add almond oil, powdered sugar, and vanilla. Chill in freezer for 15 minutes, or until mixture is cool but hasn't begun to set.

3. Using hand mixer or whisk, add ice water and nonfat milk powder to a chilled bowl; beat until peaks start to form. Add gelatin mixture to whipped milk; continue to whip for 10 minutes until stiffer peaks begin to form. This whipped topping will keep several days in refrigerator. Whip again to reintroduce more air into topping before serving.

Chocolate Cheesecake Mousse

NUTRITIONAL ANALYSIS (per serving):

Calories: 83   Protein: 3g   Carbohydrates: 7g   Fat: 5g   Saturated Fat: 2g   Cholesterol: 9mg
Sodium: 47mg   Fiber: 0g   PCF Ratio: 13-32-55   Exchange Approx.: ½ Skim Milk, 1 Fat

INGREDIENTS | SERVES 4

1 tablespoon semisweet chocolate chips

¾ cup Mock Whipped Cream
(Chapter 19)

1 ounce cream cheese

1½ teaspoons cocoa

1 teaspoon vanilla

1. Put chocolate chips and 1 tablespoon of Mock Whipped Cream in microwave-safe bowl; microwave on high for 15 seconds.

2. Add cream cheese; microwave on high for another 15 seconds. Whip mixture until well blended and chocolate chips are melted.

3. Stir in cocoa and vanilla; fold in remaining Mock Whipped Cream. Chill until ready to serve.

Nonfat Whipped Milk Base

NUTRITIONAL ANALYSIS (per recipe):

Calories: 290   Carbohydrates: 42g   Protein: 28g   Fat: 1g   Saturated Fat: 0g   Cholesterol: 11mg
Sodium: 310mg   Fiber: 0g   PCF Ratio: 39-59-2   Exchange Approx.: 2 Skim Milks, 1 Carbohydrate

INGREDIENTS | YIELDS ABOUT 3 CUPS

¼ cup nonfat milk powder
⅛ cup powdered sugar
1 cup chilled skim milk, divided
1½ envelopes Knox Unflavored Gelatine

Whipping Methods

Because you don't need to whip the Whipped Milk Base until it reaches stiff peaks, you can use a blender or food processor; however, you won't be whipping as much air into the mixture if you do, so the serving sizes will be a bit smaller.

1. In chilled bowl, combine milk powder and sugar; mix until well blended. Pour ¼ cup milk and gelatin into blender; let sit for 1–2 minutes for gelatin to soften.

2. In microwave-safe container, heat remaining milk until it almost reaches boiling point, or 30–45 seconds, on high. Add milk to blender with gelatin; blend 2 minutes, or until gelatin is completely dissolved. Chill for 15 minutes, or until mixture is cool but gelatin hasn't yet begun to set.

3. Using hand mixer or whisk, beat until doubled in size. (It won't form stiff peaks like whipped cream; however, you'll notice it will get creamier in color.) Chill until ready to use in following desserts. If necessary, whip again immediately prior to folding in other ingredients.

Raspberry Yogurt Delight

NUTRITIONAL ANALYSIS (per serving):

Calories: 121   Protein: 6g   Carbohydrates: 18g   Fat: 3g   Saturated Fat: 2g   Cholesterol: 12mg
Sodium: 74mg   Fiber: 1g   PCF Ratio: 19-59-22   Exchange Approx.: 1 Milk, ½ Fat

INGREDIENTS | SERVES 4; SERVING SIZE ½ CUP

1½ cups plain nonfat yogurt
2 tablespoons Splenda Granulated
4 tablespoons heavy cream
1 tablespoon Splenda Granulated
¼ cup Raspberry Sauce (Chapter 19)

1. Combine yogurt and 2 tablespoons Splenda in bowl; chill in refrigerator.

2. In separate bowl, whip heavy cream until moderately stiff; stir in 1 tablespoon Splenda.

3. To make dessert: Gently fold cream into yogurt. Spoon mixture into 4 dessert or parfait cups. Swirl 1 tablespoon prepared Raspberry Sauce into each cup and serve.

Raspberry Sauce

NUTRITIONAL ANALYSIS (per serving):

Calories: 38   Protein: 1g   Carbohydrates: 9g   Fat: 0g   Saturated Fat: 0g   Cholesterol: 0mg
Sodium: 1mg   Fiber: 3g   PCF Ratio: 5-89-6   Exchange Approx.: ½ Fruit

**INGREDIENTS | YIELDS 12 SERVINGS;
SERVING SIZE ¼ CUP**

4 cups raspberries
2 tablespoons Splenda Granulated
2 tablespoons honey
1 teaspoon corn starch
½ tablespoon lemon juice

1. Rinse berries; drain. Put in sauce pan; mash.

2. Add Splenda and honey; cook over medium heat until mixture reaches slow boil. Reduce heat; simmer another 10 minutes.

3. Strain berry juice through mesh sieve to remove seeds. Return to saucepan.

4. In separate small bowl, mix cornstarch with lemon juice until dissolved; add to strained berry juice. Bring liquid to a boil, stirring frequently until mixture thickens slightly, about 10 minutes.

5. Cool and store in refrigerator. Use as dessert topping or mixed in yogurt or pudding.

Peach Bread Pudding

NUTRITIONAL ANALYSIS (per serving):

Calories: 164 Protein: 7g Carbohydrates: 23g Fat: 5g Saturated Fat: 3g Cholesterol: 63mg
Sodium: 175mg Fiber: 2g PCF Ratio: 16-55-29 Exchange Approx.: 1 Starch, ½ Fruit, 1 Fat

INGREDIENTS | SERVES 9; SERVING SIZE: ½ CUP

Nonstick cooking spray
2 cups 1% milk
2 tablespoons butter
2 eggs
⅓ cup egg whites
1 teaspoon vanilla
2 teaspoons cinnamon
⅓ cup Splenda Brown Sugar Blend
6 slices whole-wheat bread, cubed
2 cups peaches, sliced

1. Preheat oven to 350°F. Spray 9" × 9" baking dish with nonstick cooking spray.

2. Heat milk in small saucepan; melt butter in milk. Cool.

3. In medium bowl, beat eggs, egg whites, vanilla, cinnamon, and Splenda.

4. Combine milk and egg mixture.

5. Place cubed bread in baking dish. Place sliced peaches on top of bread cubes. Pour egg mixture over bread and peaches. Bake for 40–45 minutes.

Key Lime Pie

NUTRITIONAL ANALYSIS (per serving):

Calories: 203   Protein: 4g   Carbohydrates: 29g   Fat: 8g   Saturated Fat: 4g   Cholesterol: 20mg
Sodium: 331mg   Fiber: 1g   PCF Ratio: 8-57-35   Exchange Approx.: 1½ Starches, 1½ Fats

INGREDIENTS | SERVES 10; SERVING SIZE: 1 SLICE

1 cup graham cracker crumbs
1 tablespoon Splenda Granulated
2 tablespoons butter
½ teaspoon lime zest
½ cup Splenda Granulated
6 ounces low-fat (Neufchâtel) cream cheese
1 package instant sugar-free vanilla pudding mix
½ cup 1% milk
1 cup lime juice (5–6 limes)
1 tablespoon Knox Unflavored Gelatine

1. Prepare graham cracker crust: Combine graham crumbs and 1 tablespoon Splenda. Add melted butter; mix well. Press crumbs into 9" pie plate with help of flat surface such as bottom of glass. Bake in 350°F oven for 10 minutes; remove from oven and cool.

2. In mixer or food processor, combine lime zest and ½ cup Splenda. Add cream cheese; process for 30 seconds. Add pudding mix and milk; blend well.

3. Pour ¼ cup lime juice into small measuring cup or bowl; heat in microwave for 1 minute. Add gelatine to heated juice; dissolve completely.

4. Mix dissolved gelatin in rest of lime juice. Turn on mixer or food processor; pour lime juice into mixture slowly. Process until all ingredients are well combined.

5. Pour filling into pie shell; refrigerate for 3–4 hours before serving. If desired, top with Mock Whipped Cream (Chapter 19).

Fall Fruit with Yogurt Sauce

NUTRITIONAL ANALYSIS (per serving):

Calories: 126   Protein: 3g   Carbohydrates: 26g   Fat: 3g   Saturated Fat: 1g   Cholesterol: 2mg
Sodium: 48mg   Fiber: 3g   PCF Ratio: 10-72-19   Exchange Approx.: 1 Fruit, ½ Milk

INGREDIENTS | SERVES 8; SERVING SIZE: ½ CUP

2 cups apples, cubed
1½ cups red seedless grapes, halved
1½ cup pears, cubed
2 teaspoons lemon juice
8 ounces light vanilla yogurt
1 teaspoon lemon juice
1 tablespoon honey
¼ cup walnuts, chopped

1. Combine apples, grapes, and pears in medium bowl. Drizzle 1 teaspoon lemon juice over fruit to prevent turning brown.

2. In small bowl, combine yogurt, 1 teaspoon lemon juice, and honey.

3. Portion ½ cup fruit per serving. Spoon yogurt dressing over fruit and top with chopped walnuts.

Fruit Compote

Calories: 117   Protein: 1g   Carbohydrates: 24g   Fat: 2g   Saturated Fat: 1g   Cholesterol: 3mg
Sodium: 29mg   Fiber: 3g   PCF Ratio: 3-80-17   Exchange Approx.: 1½ Fruits, ½ Fat

INGREDIENTS | SERVES 4; SERVING SIZE: ½ CUP

2 cups apples, chopped

2 tablespoons dried cranberries

6 dried apricots, diced

¼ teaspoon cinnamon

2 tablespoons water

1 tablespoon brandy (optional; if not used, add additional 3 tablespoons water)

1 tablespoon walnuts, finely chopped

1. Combine apples, cranberries, apricots, cinnamon, water, and brandy in small saucepan.

2. Cook over medium heat until apples are softened, about 10 minutes. Remove from heat and cover 5 minutes. Stir in walnuts before serving.

Strawberry Ricotta Pie

NUTRITIONAL ANALYSIS (per serving):

Calories: 238   Protein: 10g   Carbohydrates: 27g   Fat: 10g   Saturated Fat: 5g   Cholesterol: 86mg
Sodium: 183mg   Fiber: 1g   PCF Ratio: 18-45-37   Exchange Approx.: 1 Starch, 1 Lean Meat, 2 Fats

INGREDIENTS | SERVES 8; SERVING SIZE: 1 SLICE

2 cups part-skim ricotta cheese

1 cup graham cracker crumbs

1 tablespoon Splenda Granulated

2 tablespoons butter

2 eggs, separated

1 teaspoon lemon extract

2 tablespoons honey

¼ cup Splenda Granulated

¼ cup egg whites

¼ teaspoon cream of tartar

2 cups strawberries, sliced

1 tablespoon cornstarch

2 tablespoons Splenda Granulated

1 tablespoon lemon juice

1 teaspoon balsamic vinegar

1. Place ricotta cheese in fine mesh strainer lined with coffee filter; allow excess water to drain from cheese for 2–3 hours.

2. Prepare graham cracker crust: Combine graham crumbs and 1 tablespoon Splenda. Add melted butter; mix well. Press crumbs into 9" pie plate with help of flat surface such as bottom of glass. Bake in 350°F oven for 10 minutes; remove from oven and cool.

3. Prepare pie filling: In medium bowl, mix ricotta cheese, egg yolks, lemon extract, honey, and ¼ cup Splenda.

4. In mixer bowl, beat egg whites (2 separated plus ¼ cup additional egg whites) with cream of tartar until soft peaks begin to form. Gently fold egg whites into ricotta mixture. Turn into pie shell; bake at 350°F for 45 minutes, or until mixture is set and top is golden brown. Remove to wire rack and cool completely.

5. Prepare glaze: In medium saucepan, combine strawberries, cornstarch, and Splenda until dry ingredients have coated strawberries. Add lemon juice and balsamic vinegar; cook over medium heat, stirring constantly. Cook mixture for 5–7 minutes, or until cornstarch liquid is clear and gently bubbling. Cool.

6. Spread cooled strawberry glaze on top of cooled pie. Chill until ready to serve.

Summer Fruit Cobbler

NUTRITIONAL ANALYSIS (per serving):

Calories: 152   Protein: 3g   Carbohydrates: 26g   Fat: 5g   Saturated Fat: 0g   Cholesterol: 0mg
Sodium: 248mg   Fiber: 4g   PCF Ratio: 8-65-27   Exchange Approx.: ½ Starch, ½ Fruit, 1 Fat

INGREDIENTS | SERVES 8; SERVING SIZE: ½ CUP

Nonstick cooking spray
1½ cups raspberries
1½ cups peaches, peeled and sliced
1 cup strawberries, sliced
¼ cup sugar
1 tablespoon Splenda
2 tablespoons whole-wheat pastry flour
1 teaspoon cinnamon
¾ cup whole-wheat pastry flour
1 tablespoon sugar
1½ teaspoons baking powder
½ teaspoon salt
2½ tablespoons canola oil
2 tablespoons milk
2 tablespoons egg whites

1. Preheat oven to 350°F. Spray 9" × 9" square baking pan with nonstick cooking spray. Put fruit in bottom of baking dish.

2. In small bowl, mix sugar, Splenda, 2 tablespoons flour, and cinnamon; sprinkle evenly over fruit.

3. In small bowl, sift together ¾ cup flour, 1 tablespoon sugar, baking powder, and salt. Add oil, milk, and egg whites; stir quickly until just mixed.

4. Drop dough by spoonfuls over fruit. If desired, loosely spread dough over fruit. Bake for 25–30 minutes, until dough is golden brown.

Fun Fruits

Any combination of fresh fruit will work well with this recipe. You will need a total of 4 cups of fruit. Fruit suggestions include blueberries, blackberries, peaches, mangoes, or plums. Keep in mind that nutritional analysis will vary somewhat with different fruit combinations.

Baked Pear Crisp

NUTRITIONAL ANALYSIS (per serving):

Calories: 200   Protein: 2g   Carbohydrates: 42g   Fat: 4g   Saturated Fat: 2g   Cholesterol: 8mg
Sodium: 53mg   Fiber: 3g   PCF Ratio: 3-82-15   Exchange Approx.: 1 Fruit, 1 Fat, 1 Starch

INGREDIENTS | SERVES 4; SERVING SIZE: ½ CUP

2 pears
2 tablespoons frozen unsweetened pineapple juice concentrate
1 teaspoon vanilla extract
1 teaspoon rum
1 tablespoon butter
⅛ cup Ener-G Brown Rice Flour
⅓ cup firmly packed brown sugar
½ cup oat bran flakes

1. Preheat oven to 375°F. Treat 9" × 13" baking dish or large flat casserole dish with nonstick cooking spray. Core and cut up pears; place in baking dish. (Except for any bruised spots, it's okay to leave skins on.)

2. In glass measuring cup, microwave frozen juice concentrate for 1 minute. Stir in vanilla and rum; pour over pears.

3. Using same measuring cup, microwave butter 30–40 seconds, until melted; set aside.

4. Toss remaining ingredients in bowl, being careful not to crush cereal. Spread uniformly over pears; dribble melted butter over top. Bake for 35 minutes, or until mixture is bubbling and top is just beginning to brown. Serve hot or cold.

Baked Pumpkin Custard

NUTRITIONAL ANALYSIS (per serving):

Calories: 130   Protein: 7g   Carbohydrates: 23g   Fat: 2g   Saturated Fat: 1g   Cholesterol: 63mg
Sodium: 89mg   Fiber: 2g   PCF Ratio: 20-68-12   Exchange Approx.: 1 Milk, 1 Vegetable, ½ Fat

INGREDIENTS | SERVES 6; SERVING SIZE: ½ CUP

2 cups solid pack or mashed cooked pumpkin

¼ cup sugar

⅓ cup Splenda Granulated

2 teaspoons cinnamon

½ teaspoon ginger

⅛ teaspoon cloves

2 eggs, slightly beaten

¼ cup egg whites

12 ounces evaporated skim milk

Pumpkin Pie

If using this recipe for pumpkin pie, pour filling in prepared pie shell and bake in a 350°F oven for 40–45 minutes, or until filling is set. The nutritional analysis per serving is: Calories: 244; Protein: 8g; Fat: 9g; Saturated fat: 3g; Cholesterol: 63mg; Carbohydrate: 33g; Sodium: 206mg; PCF ratio: 13-33-54. Exchange Approx.: 1 Starch, 1 Milk, 1 Vegetable, 3 Fats.

1. Preheat oven to 350°F.

2. Mix together pumpkin, sugar, Splenda, cinnamon, ginger, and cloves. Add eggs, egg whites, and evaporated milk; whisk until well blended.

3. Pour into 6 custard cups or 1½ quart casserole dish. Set cups or casserole in large baking pan; put pan on rack in oven and pour hot water into pan to within ½" of top of custard.

4. Bake in custard cups for 40–45 minutes, 1½ quart casserole for 60–70 minutes, until knife inserted in center comes out clean. Remove immediately from hot water. Serve warm or chilled.

Strawberry Rhubarb Cobbler

NUTRITIONAL ANALYSIS (per serving):

Calories: 138   Protein: 3g   Carbohydrates: 27g   Fat: 3g   Saturated Fat: 0g   Cholesterol: 7mg
Sodium: 223mg   Fiber: 3g   PCF Ratio: 7-76-17   Exchange Approx.: ½ Starch, ½ Fruit, ½ Fat

INGREDIENTS | SERVES 9; SERVING SIZE: ½ CUP

Nonstick cooking spray
4 cups rhubarb, chopped
2 cups strawberries, thickly sliced
¼ teaspoon lemon zest
⅓ cup sugar
¼ cup Splenda Granulated
2 tablespoons cornstarch
2 tablespoons water
¾ cup whole-wheat pastry flour
1 tablespoon sugar
¼ teaspoon ginger
1½ teaspoons baking powder
½ teaspoon salt
2½ tablespoons canola oil
2 tablespoons milk
2 tablespoons egg whites

1. Preheat oven to 375°F. Spray 8" × 8" baking dish with nonstick cooking spray.

2. In mixing bowl, combine rhubarb, strawberries, lemon zest, sugar, and Splenda. Dissolve cornstarch in water. Pour over fruit; stir to coat. Place in prepared baking dish; set aside.

3. In small bowl, sift together flour, sugar, ginger, baking powder, and salt. Add oil, milk, and egg whites; stir quickly until just mixed.

4. Drop dough by spoonfuls over fruit. If desired, loosely spread dough over fruit. Bake for 25–30 minutes, until dough is golden brown.

Cranberry Pecan Biscotti

NUTRITIONAL ANALYSIS (per serving):

Calories: 98   Protein: 3g   Carbohydrates: 15g   Fat: 3g   Saturated Fat: 1g   Cholesterol: 20mg
Sodium: 39mg   Fiber: 2g   PCF Ratio: 10-59-3   Exchange Approx.: 1 Starch, ½ Fat

INGREDIENTS | YIELDS 30 BISCOTTI; SERVING SIZE: 1 BISCOTTI

4 tablespoons sweet butter, softened
½ cup sugar
½ cup Splenda Granulated
2 eggs
½ cup egg whites
1 teaspoon vanilla extract
1 teaspoon lemon zest
2½ cups all-purpose flour
⅛ teaspoon salt
½ teaspoon baking powder
½ cup pecans, chopped
½ cup dried cranberries

Exchange List

Food exchange lists can be an important part of arriving at individualized meal plans. To see a full list of foods with their exchange value visit *www.mayoclinic.com/health/diabetes-diet/DA00077*.

1. Preheat oven to 350°F. In medium bowl, beat butter, sugar, Splenda, eggs, egg whites, vanilla, and lemon zest until smooth.

2. In separate bowl, sift flour, salt, and baking powder. Add dry ingredients to liquid ingredients; mix well. Add pecans and cranberries. Chill dough for 1–2 hours, which makes it easier to handle.

3. Divide dough in ½; shape each ½ into slightly flattened 3" × 9" loaf. Place loaves on greased cookie sheet; bake for 25 minutes.

4. Remove from oven; when cooled enough to handle, cut into ½" slices. Lay out slices on cookie sheet and return to oven for 20 minutes until toasted on bottom.

5. Remove from oven; turn over and bake for 15 minutes until other side is toasted as well. Remove from oven and cool on wire rack.

Your 10-Week Plan to Kick Pre-Diabetes!

The 10-week Plan to Kick Pre-Diabetes is designed to help you set modest goals and put what you have learned into practice. Each week has a healthy lifestyle theme along with two suggested goals to help you achieve success.

Week 1: Check Your Portions

Portion control is everything, even when you choose healthy foods! If you eat large portions, you will have trouble controlling your calories. One simple approach to controlling portions is to use the plate method. The concept is designed to help you put together healthy meals in correct portions and distribute carbohydrates evenly in meals. Using the plate method at lunch and dinner, fill half of your plate with vegetables, one-quarter of the plate with starches, and one-quarter of the plate with meat or meat substitute. A serving of milk and fruit are also added to the meal.

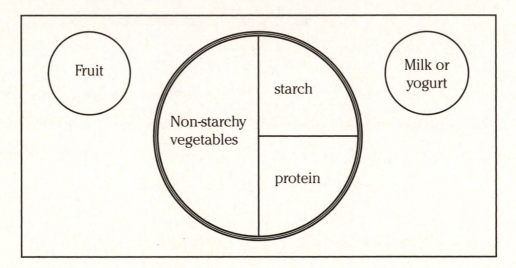

YOUR GOALS FOR WEEK 1

- Give the plate method a try as a means to reduce portion sizes.
- For several days, measure or weigh your food so you can see just how much you are eating.

Week 2: Eat More Vegetables and Fruit Every Day

The recommendation to eat five to nine servings of fruit and vegetables every day sounds like a lot of food, but once you know how to incorporate these foods into you plan it becomes easy. Why that many servings? Because fruit and vegetables are nutrient-dense foods with high fiber and lower calories.

- Take two pieces of fruit from home each day to have for a mid-meal snack or with lunch.
- Keep raw vegetables washed, cut-up, and ready to eat for quick snacks or salads. If they are there, you will eat them!

Week 3: Get Walking!

Start walking, even if you are only able to manage a few minutes at a time. No matter how long you are able to walk, doing it consistently is most important. Aim for walking most days of the week. Make sure that you have comfortable walking shoes or sneakers.

YOUR GOALS FOR WEEK 3

- Walk for as long as you are comfortably able to. Keep a written record of when and how long you are walking.
- Wear a pedometer so you can track how many steps you take each day. Use the number of steps you take as a motivator to help you increase it each day.

Week 4: Switch to Whole Grains

Begin to switch out the white flour and white grain products in your kitchen for whole grain foods. Whole grains provide more fiber and nutrients, and have less impact on your blood glucose. Look for products that list whole grain flour, rather than enriched flour as one of the first ingredients.

YOUR GOALS FOR WEEK 4

- Add whole grain pasta or brown rice to a favorite dish or in combination with vegetables or beans.
- Purchase a new whole grain food that you haven't used before and try it as a replacement for rice, pasta, or potatoes. Some suggestions: quinoa, kasha, or bulgur.

Week 5: Manage Your Stress

Take stress seriously and find ways to reduce it. Chronic stress can wreak havoc on health and well being by lowering your immunity and making you more susceptible to many types of illness. You are working on ways to halt pre-diabetes in its tracks; don't let stress derail you!

YOUR GOALS FOR WEEK 5
- Add stretching exercises, meditation, or deep breathing exercises to your daily routine.
- Allow yourself some downtime from the daily grind each day. Make this time for yourself by choosing a relaxing activity that that you enjoy.

Week 6: Get Adequate Sleep

Insufficient sleep can have a negative impact on your health. New research has shown that poor quality sleep on a regular basis can contribute to insulin resistance, metabolic syndrome, and diabetes. Just what you are trying to avoid!

YOUR GOALS FOR WEEK 6
- Even if you are very busy or have a demanding schedule resist the urge to skimp on sleep. Make enough time to get seven to eight hours of sleep each night.
- Develop good sleeping habits by rising and retiring about the same time each day. Avoid distractions such as the television at times when you should be going to sleep.

Week 7: Don't Forget the Snacks

Having meals and snacks at regular times can go a long way toward controlling your appetite and blood glucose. Snacking during the day is fine, as long as you are making good choices that are low in calories and have nutritional value.

GOALS FOR WEEK 7

- When you grocery shop, buy healthy snacks to have on hand at all times. Come up with at least two new snack options this week to prevent boredom.
- If necessary, prepare snacks ahead of time, so they are always ready to go, e.g., cut up vegetables, pre-measure nuts into individual containers/baggies, etc.

Week 8: Ramp up Your Exercise

You may have started an exercise plan several weeks ago, but it's time to take it up a notch. This is important because exercising the same muscles or at the same intensity all of the time will eventually stall you efforts at weight loss.

GOALS FOR WEEK 8

- Turn your moderate walk into a brisk walk. Step up the pace of your walk and add additional steps by using your pedometer to measure your progress.
- Add a few flexibility or weight bearing exercises to your routine in addition to the walking.

Week 9: Change Your Food Behaviors

Negative food habits are not always easy to change. Make a conscious effort to correct eating habits that cause you to get off track.

GOALS FOR WEEK 9

- Slow down when you eat. Fast eating or mindless eating can cause you to eat too much food before you realize that you've had enough to eat. Place your fork down between each bite and allow more time to eat your meal or snack.
- Drink plenty of water. Take a water bottle with you wherever you go, set one on your desk at work, or find ways to remind yourself to drink more water. Most people need about 64 ounces of fluid a day; make most of it water!

Week 10: Progress Check—Putting It All Together

Monitor your overall progress by looking at how well you have done with various aspects of your plan.

GOALS FOR WEEK 10

- Make a list of all of the things you have been able to achieve, as well as the goals that still need work.
- Seeing in writing all that you have accomplished is very satisfying and motivates you to keep going. Congratulate and reward yourself for a job well done!

APPENDIX B

Resources

As you learn more about diabetes, you may have more questions or want to find out additional information. The following resources provide a wealth of information regarding diabetes in general, as well as diets, forums, and frequently asked questions.

Online Sources for Diabetes Information

American Dietetic Association

⌐ *www.eatright.org*

The American Dietetic Association is the world's largest organization of food and nutrition professionals. This site provides nutrition information and resources on a variety of topics and includes a tool to find a dietitian in your area.

American Diabetes Association

⌐ *www.diabetes.org*

This site, maintained by the recognized authority on diabetes, is dedicated to providing up-to-date information regarding medications and diabetes research findings.

Ask the Dietitian

⌐ *www.dietitian.com*

Joanne Larsen, MS, RD, LD, maintains this site. You can use it to post specific diet-related questions or read the answers to questions from other visitors.

Changing Life with Diabetes

⌐ *www.changingdiabetes-us.com*

An interactive website with menu-planning tools and information about different types of insulin.

dLife

⌐ *www.dLife.com*

An interactive diabetes website that includes diabetes information, tips for healthy eating, a recipe bank, and a diabetic community.

National Institute of Diabetes & Digestive & Kidney Disease

🖰 *www.niddk.nih.gov*

> Site for general diabetes information, where brochures and articles can be downloaded.

The U.S. National Library of Medicine and National Institute of Health

🖰 *www.nlm.nih.gov/medlineplus/diabetes.html*

> This site has research, references, interactive tutorial, consumer materials, and guidebooks to download or order online.

Online Sources for Ingredients and Equipment

The quality of the foods you prepare is based on the quality of the ingredients you use; that's elementary. The equipment you use can make a difference, too. Even if you don't have a gourmet grocery or cooking supply store nearby, you don't have to forego using out-of-the-ordinary ingredients or products you've been wanting to try. Chances are you can order them online through one of these sites.

Ancient Harvest

🖰 *www.quinoa.net*

Barilla Plus Pasta

🖰 *www.barillaus.com*

Bob's Red Mill

🖰 *www.bobsredmill.com*

Cabot Cheese

🖰 *www.cabotcheese.coop*

Chef's Catalog

🖰 *www.chefscatalog.com*

King Arthur Flours

🖰 *www.kingarthurflours.com*

McCormick Spice

🖰 *www.mccormick.com*

MexGrocer.com

🖰 *www.mexgrocer.com*

Mrs. Dash

🖰 *www.mrsdash.com*

Visit these sites to find a location near you:

Local Harvest
🖱 *www.localharvest.org*

Use this website to find farmers' markets, family farms, and other sources of sustainably grown food in your area, where you can buy produce, grass-fed meats, and many other locally grown foods.

Trader Joe's
🖱 *www.traderjoes.com*

Whole Foods Market
🖱 *www.wholefoodsmarket.com*

For an online food exchange list:

The Mayo Clinic
🖱 *www.mayoclinic.com/health/diabetes-diet/DA00077*

Standard U.S./Metric Measurement Conversions

VOLUME CONVERSIONS

U.S. Volume Measure	Metric Equivalent
⅛ teaspoon	0.5 milliliters
¼ teaspoon	1 milliliters
½ teaspoon	2 milliliters
1 teaspoon	5 milliliters
½ tablespoon	7 milliliters
1 tablespoon (3 teaspoons)	15 milliliters
2 tablespoons (1 fluid ounce)	30 milliliters
¼ cup (4 tablespoons)	60 milliliters
⅓ cup	90 milliliters
½ cup (4 fluid ounces)	125 milliliters
⅔ cup	160 milliliters
¾ cup (6 fluid ounces)	180 milliliters
1 cup (16 tablespoons)	250 milliliters
1 pint (2 cups)	500 milliliters
1 quart (4 cups)	1 liter (about)

WEIGHT CONVERSIONS

U.S. Weight Measure	Metric Equivalent
½ ounce	15 grams
1 ounce	30 grams
2 ounces	60 grams
3 ounces	85 grams
¼ pound (4 ounces)	115 grams
½ pound (8 ounces)	225 grams
¾ pound (12 ounces)	340 grams
1 pound (16 ounces)	454 grams

OVEN TEMPERATURE CONVERSIONS

Degrees Fahrenheit	Degrees Celsius
200 degrees F	100 degrees C
250 degrees F	120 degrees C
275 degrees F	140 degrees C
300 degrees F	150 degrees C
325 degrees F	160 degrees C
350 degrees F	180 degrees C
375 degrees F	190 degrees C
400 degrees F	200 degrees C
425 degrees F	220 degrees C
450 degrees F	230 degrees C

BAKING PAN SIZES

American	Metric
8 x 1½ inch round baking pan	20 x 4 cm cake tin
9 x 1½ inch round baking pan	23 x 3.5 cm cake tin
1 x 7 x 1½ inch baking pan	28 x 18 x 4 cm baking tin
13 x 9 x 2 inch baking pan	30 x 20 x 5 cm baking tin
2 quart rectangular baking dish	30 x 20 x 3 cm baking tin
15 x 10 x 2 inch baking pan	30 x 25 x 2 cm baking tin (Swiss roll tin)
9 inch pie plate	22 x 4 or 23 x 4 cm pie plate
7 or 8 inch springform pan	18 or 20 cm springform or loose bottom cake tin
9 x 5 x 3 inch loaf pan	23 x 13 x 7 cm or 2 lb narrow loaf or pate tin
1½ quart casserole	1.5 litre casserole
2 quart casserole	2 litre casserole

Index

We Have
EVERYTHING®
on Anything!

With more than 19 million copies sold, **the Everything® series** has become one of America's favorite resources for solving problems, learning new skills, and organizing lives. Our brand is not only recognizable—it's also welcomed.

The series is a hand-in-hand partner for people who are ready to tackle new subjects—like you!

For more information on the Everything® series, please visit *www.adamsmedia.com*

The Everything® list spans a wide range of subjects, with more than 500 titles covering 25 different categories:

Business	History	Reference
Careers	Home Improvement	Religion
Children's Storybooks	Everything Kids	Self-Help
Computers	Languages	Sports & Fitness
Cooking	Music	Travel
Crafts and Hobbies	New Age	Wedding
Education/Schools	Parenting	Writing
Games and Puzzles	Personal Finance	
Health	Pets	